Groundwater Recharge with Reclaimed Water

An Epidemiologic Assessment in Los Angeles County, 1987–1991

Elizabeth M. Sloss

Sandra A. Geschwind

Daniel F. McCaffrey

Beate R. Ritz

Prepared for the Water Replenishment District of Southern California

RAND

CONTENTS

TABLES

The epidemiologic study reported here investigated the rate of health outcomes in the Montebello Forebay region of Los Angeles County from 1987 to 1991, almost 30 years after some reclaimed water was first used to replenish the groundwater supply in the basin. Previous epidemiologic studies concluded that the level of reclaimed water used for recharge in the Montebello Forebay from 1962 to 1980 had no detectable impact on human health (Nellor et al., 1984; Frerichs et al., 1981, 1982, 1983). The current research was undertaken to update the results of these studies.

The percentage of reclaimed water in residential water supplies was estimated for the 66 water system service areas in the Montebello Forebay for 1960 through 1991 by Bookman-Edmonston Engineering, Inc. (Bookman-Edmonston Engineering, Inc., 1993a). Eight of these service areas did not receive any reclaimed water during this time period. In the other service areas, the maximum percentage of reclaimed water over the 30-year period was estimated to be between 0 and 4 percent in 14 systems, between 5 and 19 percent in 19 systems, and between 20 and 31 percent in 25 systems. For most systems, the percentage of reclaimed water increased over the 30-year period. For the purposes of this study, each census tract receiving reclaimed water was allocated to one of five exposure categories based on the percentage of reclaimed water in its supplies.

As of 1990, approximately 900,000 people living in the Montebello Forebay area of Los Angeles County received some reclaimed water in their household supply. These people account for more than 10 percent of the population of Los Angeles County. To compare rates of disease and death, a control area with similar demographic and socioeconomic characteristics but not receiving any reclaimed water was selected. The control area includes about 700,000 people in three locations within Los Angeles County: parts of the Montebello Forebay, Pomona, and the northeastern San Fernando Valley.

Using an ecologic study design, a hypothesis of an association between reclaimed water and a broad range of biologically plausible health outcomes was tested. Existing data on cancer incidence (1987–1991 cancer registry records), mortality (1989–1991 death certificates), and infectious disease (1989–1990 reports to the health department) were analyzed in conjunction with population counts from the 1990 Census. Rates of the health outcomes were compared between the reclaimed water and matched control areas. Poisson regression methods were used to generate rate ratios and 95 percent confidence intervals.

This epidemiologic study concludes that almost 30 years after groundwater recharge with some reclaimed water began, the rates of cancer, mortality, and infectious disease are similar in both the area of Los Angeles County receiving some reclaimed water and a control area not receiving reclaimed water. Rates of these health outcomes are also similar in areas receiving higher and lower percentages of reclaimed water. The analysis included routinely collected data on cancer incidence (all cancers and cancer of the bladder, colon, esophagus, kidney, liver, pancreas, rectum, and stomach), mortality (deaths due to all causes, heart disease, stroke, all cancer, and the eight specific cancer sites), and infectious diseases (giardia, hepatitis A, salmonella, shigella, and several less common diseases). There were few instances in which rates of disease or death were significantly higher in areas receiving reclaimed water than in the control area. Regions with less reclaimed water tended to have higher rates of adverse health outcomes than regions with more reclaimed water, leading to the conclusion that the observed higher rates were probably due either to chance or to other unmeasured factors unrelated to reclaimed water exposure. A significantly higher incidence rate of liver cancer was observed in the area with the highest percentage of reclaimed water. Because there is no biologic or epidemiologic evidence to suggest a relationship between reclaimed water and liver cancer, this result is most likely explained by factors unrelated to reclaimed water or by chance occurrence.

The limitations of epidemiologic methods make drawing definitive conclusions about the effect of reclaimed water on health difficult. Personal characteristics that might affect disease rates such as smoking, alcohol consumption, and occupational exposure were assumed to be equal in the reclaimed water and control areas, but could not be controlled in the analysis. If the distribution of these factors differs substantially between the reclaimed water and control areas, the pattern of results may be attributable to these differences or other uncontrolled factors. In addition, actual exposure to reclaimed water may differ from that estimated because of time spent away from home and consumption of bottled water and other beverages. Finally, the high population mobility in Los Angeles County may make detecting an effect more difficult. Despite its limitations, the results of this epidemiologic study do not provide evidence that reclaimed water has an adverse effect on health.

We would like to acknowledge the efforts of many people without whom this research would not have been possible. We would like to thank Suzanne Polich and Deborah Wesley at RAND for their outstanding work in preparing the data files for analysis. Harold Morgan, Richard Anderson, and others at Bookman-Edmonston Engineering, Inc. provided RAND with the data on reclaimed water and an abundance of other water-related information. Dennis Deapen of the University of Southern California Cancer Surveillance Program arranged for RAND's use of the cancer incidence data. Hong Chen of the Los Angeles County Department of Health Services (LACDHS) assembled the mortality and infectious disease data for RAND under the direction of Larry Portigal. Nancy Austin of the State of California Department of Finance furnished RAND with data from the 1990 U.S. Census.

We would also like to acknowledge the contributions of others. We would like to thank Nancy Moore of RAND and Kenneth Cantor of the National Cancer Institute for excellent suggestions based on their reviews of an early draft. The report also incorporates the thoughtful suggestions of Rodger Baird and Margaret Nellor of the County Sanitation Districts of Los Angeles County, and Harold Morgan of Bookman-Edmonston Engineering, Inc. In addition, we appreciate the valuable suggestions made by the members of the advisory committee set up to oversee the epidemiology study, in particular Raymond Neutra of the State of California Department of Health Services and Shirley Fannin of the Los Angeles County Department of Health Services. Finally, we are grateful for the support and assistance of the Water Replenishment District of Southern California throughout this project, especially Mario Garcia (our project officer), Jeff Helsley, Assistant General Manager, and Fred Cardenas, General Manager.

Some areas in Southern California have chosen to replenish the groundwater with water from other sources. The process of replacing water in underground aquifers is called groundwater recharge (Nellor et al., 1984).

This study examines the possible effects on human health of using reclaimed water to recharge a groundwater basin. The use of reclaimed water for groundwater recharge began in the Montebello Forebay region of south-central Los Angeles County in 1962. Over the past 30 years, the volume of reclaimed water used to replenish the Montebello Forebay basin has increased from 12,000 acre-feet per year in 1962 to 50,000 acre-feet per year in the mid-1980s. Other water sources have also been used to recharge the basin, including local stormwater runoff and imported surface water from the Colorado River and State Water Project (Nellor et al., 1984).

Wastewater Reuse

Throughout history, man has discharged waste matter into bodies of water. With small numbers of humans and large volumes of water, nature degraded the waste without harming the environment. As the waste volume increased, the delicate balance in these waters shifted, leading to pollution. Now, in many places in the United States, reclaiming water for reuse is a carefully monitored treatment process.

Currently, wastewater is reused in several ways throughout the United States. *Direct reuse* consists of treated wastewater that is delivered to the user directly by pipe or through a reservoir. In the United States, direct reuse is restricted to nonpotable uses such as industrial processes, recreational facilities, and irrigation. Untreated household wastewater (other than toilet wastewater), called "gray water," is used for domestic irrigation and toilet flushing. All of these methods of reusing water are called *intentional direct reuse for nonpotable purposes* (Blanton, 1992).

When treated and untreated wastewater is returned to a river or other body of water, it is often inadvertently withdrawn from these sources for use. This type of *indirect* reuse commonly occurs in rivers. If the body of water both receives wastewater and is the source of drinking water, this unplanned and uncontrolled reuse is called *unintentional indirect reuse. Intentional indirect reuse of reclaimed wastewater for potable purposes* is a term reserved for planned groundwater recharge with extensively treated tertiary effluents from water reclamation plants (Blanton, 1992).

Intentional indirect potable reuse currently takes place at five locations in the United States (Hamann et al., 1991). One of them, the Montebello Forebay (Whittier Narrows Water Reclamation Plant) in Los Angeles County, California, is the focus of this study. Two of the other sites are also located in California: Water Factory 21 in Orange County and the Tahoe-Truckee Sanitation Agency Water Reclamation Plant in Nevada County. The remaining two sites are the Upper Occoquan Sewage Authority (UOSA) Water Reclamation Plant in Fairfax County, Virginia, and the Fred Hervey Water Reclamation Plant in El Paso, Texas.

Residents of other areas of the United States may be exposed to much higher percentages of reclaimed water in their household supplies than those areas with intentional indirect reuse of reclaimed water (Robeck et al., 1987). Some river water may contain much higher percentages of "reclaimed water" than water from groundwater basins replenished with some reclaimed water. For example, residents of Cincinnati and New Orleans use river water downstream from major drainage basins that collect from numerous municipal and industrial outflows. Although such water may not be reclaimed using a formal treatment process and may not be reused in an "intentional" manner, it is nonetheless reclaimed and reused water.

Treatment of Reclaimed Water

Reclaimed water arises from municipal wastewater that has been used in households, workplaces, and industries. This wastewater flows from its point of use through clay or concrete pipes to treatment plants. The process used to treat the wastewater at these plants essentially duplicates and accelerates what occurs in nature. A multistep treatment process is used to convert the wastewater to reuseable water (Figure 1.1).

In a process similar to other sewage treatment plants, the water reclamation plants in Los Angeles County start their wastewater treatment with primary and secondary treatment. The wastewater is transported from the sewer lines into a long concrete tank for its primary treatment. During primary treatment, sand, gravel, and other inorganic materials are allowed to settle out in tanks (sedimentation). Secondary treatment depends on biological processes to digest much of the remaining organic waste. Bacteria and other microorganisms break down the organic material in an

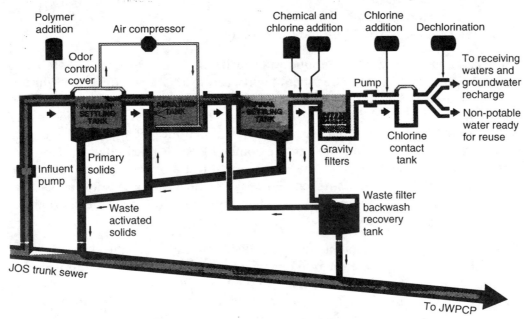

SOURCE: County Sanitation Districts of Los Angeles County.

Figure 1.1—Treatment Process in Los Angeles County Sanitation Districts' Water Reclamation Plants

aerated tank to produce harmless by-products such as carbon dioxide and water. After this process is completed, the bacteria-laden sludge is separated from the remaining liquid by settling. During primary and secondary treatment, suspended solids are reduced by about 90 percent. Secondary treatment is effective in reducing the number of viruses and bacteria, and removing metals (through sludge) and organic chemicals (through biodegradation).

The next stage of treatment at the water reclamation plants goes beyond what sewage treatment plants normally provide. This stage, called tertiary treatment, consists of mono- or dual-media filtration at Los Angeles County reclamation plants. The filtration is followed by disinfection through chlorination. Treatment with chlorine is essential for controlling infectious agents in the reclaimed wastewater.

Very few halogenated organic compounds occur in reclaimed water from Los Angeles County plants. Halogenated organics (e.g., trihalomethanes) are formed during a reaction between chlorine and organic material in the water, and have been associated with health risks in some studies (Robeck et al., 1987). The potential to form such compounds depends largely on the absence of ammonia. Because the effluent from the Los Angeles County reclamation plants contains ammonia, few halogenated organics are formed. To prevent production of halogenated organics after leaving the treatment plant, the water is dechlorinated.

Assuming the wastewater treatment plants perform reliably, Robeck et al. (1987) claim that extensively treated wastewater might well be of better quality than many surface waters commonly used as sources of drinking water.

Reclaimed Water in the Montebello Forebay

The reclaimed water used for groundwater recharge in the Montebello Forebay is currently produced by three treatment plants. From 1962 until 1973, the Whittier Narrows Water Reclamation Plant (WRP) was the sole provider of reclaimed water in the form of disinfected secondary effluent. In 1973, the San Jose Creek Water Reclamation Plant began supplying secondary effluent for recharge. Some surplus effluent from a third treatment plant, the Pomona WRP, is released to the San Jose Wash, which ultimately flows to the San Gabriel River and becomes an incidental source for recharge in the Montebello Forebay. In 1978, all three WRPs added tertiary treatment with mono- or dual-media filtration and chlorination/dechlorination to their treatment regime.

After leaving the reclamation plants, the reclaimed water is conveyed to spreading areas whereby it can be delivered to one of several destinations. Effluent from the Whittier Narrows WRP can be delivered to the Rio Hondo spreading grounds from either of two discharge points. Alternatively, Whittier Narrows effluent is carried via pipeline from the plant to the San Gabriel River. San Jose Creek WRP effluent usually is conveyed through a pipeline to the San Gabriel River. From this point, water can either be released for spreading in the unlined San Gabriel River channel or in the adjacent spreading grounds. Effluent from the San Jose Creek WRP also can be released to the San Jose Wash and then delivered either to the San Gabriel River or conveyed across the Whittier Narrows to the Rio Hondo where it can be diverted into the Rio Hondo spreading grounds.

The reclaimed water is blended with other sources of water in the underground aquifers. The regulatory agency responsible for overseeing the spreading operations (the Regional Water Quality Control Board) allows blending of reclaimed water with other sources as the reclaimed water moves underground through the aquifers. There are no regulatory provisions that require blending to take place at the surface prior to groundwater recharge. Only a portion of recharged waters can consist of reclaimed water, with limitations calculated based on both annual and three-year running averages. No more than 50 percent of recharged water in any one year can consist of reclaimed water. On a running three-year-average basis, no more than 35 percent of total recharge to the Montebello Forebay can consist of reclaimed water. In actual volumes, reclaimed water can amount to no more than 60,000 acre-feet annually and no more than 150,000 acre-feet over a running three-year period. The dilution resulting from this blending step is important in reducing the concentration of any contaminants in any of the sources used for recharge (Nellor et al., 1984).

In the process of groundwater recharge, the water percolates through an unsaturated zone of soil ranging in average thickness of about 10 to 40 feet before reaching the groundwater table. The process of "surface spreading"[1] takes place in several areas, including two areas of spreading ground facilities (San Gabriel River and Rio Hondo) and in the unlined San Gabriel River channel. These areas together cover some 700 wetted acres of land in the Montebello Forebay recharge operation. The usual spreading schedule consists of a repeated 21-day cycle of flooding and drying. The cycle consists of five days of flooding during which water is piped into the basins and maintained at a constant depth. The flow is then discontinued, followed by 16 days during which the basins are allowed to drain and dry out. This cycle of wet and dry maintains the proper conditions for the percolation process (Crook et al, 1990; Nellor et al., 1984). During percolation, trace organic compounds are reduced substantially, primarily through biodegradation, aided somewhat by adsorption and volatilization (Nellor et al., 1984).

Regulation of Reclaimed Water Use in California

In the early 1970s, the State Water Resources Control Board (SWRCB) oversaw the development of long-range plans for water basins throughout California. These plans identified more than 30 projects entailing groundwater recharge, some of which proposed augmenting domestic water sources with reclaimed water (Crook et al., 1990). In response to these plans, the California Department of Health Services (DOHS) issued a position statement in 1973 regarding the proposed uses of reclaimed water.

---

[1] Surface spreading is a method of groundwater recharge in which the water travels from the land surface to the aquifer by infiltration and percolation through the soil. Spreading basins are the areas of land designated for surface spreading (Crook et al., 1992).

In this position statement, the DOHS outlined guidelines for use of reclaimed water, including what it considered inappropriate uses, such as direct addition of reclaimed water into domestic water supplies, and direct injection into groundwater (i.e., without percolation). As justification for these recommendations, the document cites the possibility of long-term health effects associated with organic material remaining in reclaimed water after treatment. Regarding surface spreading of reclaimed water, it stated that the use of surface spreading seems promising; the health effects of surface spreading are unknown; if recharge with reclaimed water is associated with adverse effects, groundwater basins might have to be closed; setting an "acceptable" level of reclaimed water was not possible without more information; and recharge of large basins with a relatively small volume of reclaimed water might be acceptable (Crook et al., 1990). In conclusion, the report stated that surface spreading of reclaimed water might be an option.

In 1975, three of California's state agencies—DOHS, SWRCB, and the Department of Water Resources (DWR)—formed a Consulting Panel on the Health Aspects of Wastewater Reclamation for Groundwater Recharge following the issuance of the DOHS position statement (Crook et al., 1990). The panel was supposed to recommend research related to reclaimed water aimed at two objectives. First, the research should enable the DOHS to formulate reasonable criteria for groundwater recharge with reclaimed water. Second, the recommended research should help the DWR and SWRCB to design and initiate programs that would encourage the use of reclaimed water in line with these criteria.

The Consulting Panel focused on research tasks related to groundwater recharge with reclaimed water by surface spreading. The panel recommended that studies be conducted to elucidate health effects and estimate any health risk (Crook et al., 1990). The studies should be aimed at characterizing any contaminants, exploring the toxicology, and studying the epidemiology of the exposed populations. The panel suggested that data for these studies should be derived from ongoing projects that were using reclaimed water, as well as new projects that could be conducted under more-controlled conditions.

In 1976, the DOHS wrote draft regulations for groundwater recharge with reclaimed water by surface spreading (Crook et al., 1990). The objectives of the proposed regulations were to eliminate stable organic chemicals from the water. The draft regulations specified that wastewater should undergo secondary treatment followed by carbon adsorption and percolation through 10 feet of soil. Water quality standards were proposed for reclaimed water for a number of constituents: inorganic chemicals, pesticides, radioactivity, chemical oxygen demand (COD), and total organic carbon (TOC). Separate standards were proposed for the quality of the groundwater receiving the reclaimed water. The draft regulations specified that reclaimed water could not exceed 50 percent of all water spread in a 12-month period, and that it should remain underground for one year before being pumped out. The proposed regulations also requested an effluent monitoring program, hydrogeology and spreading reports, an industrial monitoring program, contingency plans, and an ongoing program to monitor the health of populations receiving reclaimed water. The breadth of these draft regulations made the implementation of the complete set too costly and unmanageable. They were not adopted as statewide criteria, but rather were recommended as guidelines for new groundwater recharge projects (Crook et al., 1990).

These wastewater reclamation criteria were revised by the DOHS in 1978 (Crook et al., 1990). The revision targeted the quality of reclaimed water to be used to recharge aquifers for domestic water supplies, requiring that the quality "fully protect public health." DOHS also suggested that each recharge project be considered based on its individual characteristics, including treatment, quality and volume of effluent, spreading grounds, soil for percolation, hydrogeology, time in aquifer, and time to withdrawal. The criteria were also amended to require a DOHS-held public hearing prior to approval of a new project.

The pressure to use reclaimed water in Southern California heightened following the 1976–1977 drought. The recommendations of the Consulting Panel, however, deterred water officials from starting new projects or expanding existing projects. In 1978, a study of health effects related to groundwater recharge with reclaimed water was initiated by the Sanitation Districts of Los Angeles County. The so-called Health Effects Study was completed over a five-year period at a cost of $1.4 million (Crook et al., 1990). The design and results of this study are summarized in the next section.

Health Effects Study

The goal of the Health Effects Study was to compile information for health and regulatory authorities who would be making decisions about the use of reclaimed water in California. One of these decisions was whether reclaimed water for groundwater recharge in the Montebello Forebay should be maintained at the same level, increased, or decreased. The information collected during the study had two objectives: (1) to assess whether groundwater recharge with reclaimed water had affected the groundwater quality or human health in an adverse way, and (2) to compare how various water sources used for recharge affected the groundwater quality (Nellor et al., 1984).

The study's research tasks included (1) water-quality characterizations of groundwater, reclaimed water, and other recharge sources, (2) toxicological and chemical studies of the same water sources, (3) studies to determine the effect of percolation on the quality of reclaimed water, (4) hydrogeological studies to establish movement of reclaimed water within the groundwater basin, and (5) epidemiologic studies of populations living in areas serving reclaimed water. The major findings of the study are summarized below, drawing heavily from the final report by Nellor et al. (1984).

Water Quality Characterization. Groundwater and reclaimed water met all federal drinking water regulations for microorganisms and for organic and inorganic chemicals. The concentration of unregulated "health-significant" organic compounds in some samples of reclaimed water and stormwater exceeded guidelines set by the California Department of Health Services. The levels of such compounds in groundwater and imported water, however, did not exceed these limits.

The water quality characterization studies revealed that a group of nontargeted industrial organics and metabolic by-products—phthalates, solvents, and petroleum by-products—were found at a significantly higher concentration than all targeted organic compounds in both reclaimed water and stormwater. Overall, in the 1984 Health Effects Study, only about 10 percent of the organic matter contained in reclaimed water was identified.

The organic complexity of the groundwater appeared to be related to the proximity of the sampling site to industrial areas. Its trihalomethane concentration was influenced by chlorination practices at the wells. The average groundwater concentration of solvents and pesticides was below estimated carcinogenic risk levels. Industrial organics were present in all groundwater samples, leading to the conclusion that water supplies need to be protected from improper handling of chemicals, mainly improper industrial waste disposal.

Virus Sampling. No viruses were recovered from groundwater or the chlorinated tertiary effluents of the four California wastewater treatment facilities in 174 samples prepared for the study.

Trace Organics Studies. The levels of trace organic compounds in reclaimed water, imported water, and stormwater exceeded some of the "theoretical lifetime risk assessment" values from the (at the time) proposed Environmental Protection Agency (EPA) water quality criteria. The average concentrations of organic compounds in *groundwater*, however, did not exceed these values. All percolation sources—reclaimed water, stormwater, and imported water—as well as unchlorinated and chlorinated well water were analyzed for the compounds listed in Table 1.1 (Nellor et al., 1984). The organic compounds detected in well water originated in all three percolation sources and from the chlorination practices at the wells. The following compounds were detected in the sources:

Surface runoff water: tetrachloroethylene, atrazine, simazine, propazine, chlorinated phenols, phenylacetic acid, and phthalates.

Reclaimed water: methylene chloride, chloroform, trichloroethylene, tetrachloroethylene, chlorinated phenols, and phthalates.

Water imported from the Colorado River: trihalomethanes and phthalates.

Chlorination practices: trihalomethanes.

Although these compounds were above the detection limits, their levels were insignificant relative to the EPA's maximum contaminant levels, the National Academy of Sciences' "suggested no adverse response levels," and the California State Department of Health Services' "action levels" (Nellor et al., 1984).

Toxicology Studies. Water concentrates from four water treatment plants were tested with a fortified Ames Salmonella Microsome Mutagen Assay. The mutagenicity of the reclaimed water was found to be intermediate between the high mutagenicity of storm runoff and dry weather runoff and the low mutagenicity of imported Colorado River water (Robeck et al., 1987). Mammalian cell assays were performed

Table 1.1

**Compounds in Target Organic Analyses
in the Health Effects Study**

Target Compounds	
vinyl chloride	DDT
methylene chloride	dieldrin
chloroform	aldrin
bromodichloromethane	lindane
dibromochloromethane	atrazine
bromoform	simazine
carbon tetrachloride	pentachlorophenol
1,1-dichloroethane	trichlorobiphenyls (as total PCB)
1,2-dichloroethane	tetrachlorobiphenyls (as total PCB)
1,1,2-trichloroethane	trichlorobenzene (1,2,4-isomer)
trichloroethylene	trichlorophenol (2,4,6-isomer)
tetrachloroethylene	trichlorophenol (2,4,5-isomer)
chlorobenzene	bis (2-ethylhexyl) phthalate
1,4-dichlorobenzene	phenylacetic acid
1,2-dichlorobenzene	fluoranthene
benzene	phenanthrene
toluene	benzo(a)pyrene

to detect presumptive carcinogenic action. None was detected for these samples. According to chemical and biological assays, the compounds responsible for the mutagenicity may have been organic halides and epoxides. Although some compounds in these classes are known mutagens and animal carcinogens, the significance of the mutagenicity finding was limited by the lack of precise identification of the compounds. The occurrence and action of such compounds may not be limited to the Montebello Forebay recharge project. Compounds similar to these may be responsible for the low-level mutagenicity found in drinking water samples nationwide.

The possibility of interactions, and the fact that many organic substances in reclaimed water are unknown or not yet identifiable, stimulated a shift from trying to classify each single compound toxicologically to assessing the mutagenic and carcinogenic potential of concentrated samples of reclaimed water as a whole. The drawback of this procedure is that it limits the assessment of the quality of reclaimed water to that produced by a specific treatment plant at only one point in time; in fact the quality of reclaimed water might vary with treatment practices as well as with the quality of the influent water. Although the results of the Ames test have not demonstrated correlations with possible health effects in humans, this test is a useful screening tool for detecting the presence of organics capable of causing damage to genetic material (as possible carcinogens) in complex organic mixtures (Nellor et al., 1984).

Percolation Studies. A study to determine possible changes in water quality resulting from the percolation of water through soil concluded that soil percolation did not consistently remove target trace organics from reclaimed water. Organic chemicals are biotransformed by microorganisms residing in subsurface material. The rate and extent of such transformation, however, are dependent on the availability of organisms and their metabolic requirements with respect to oxygen, pH, and mineral nutrients. The adsorption capacity of soil is variable; materials introduced by repeated spreading of treated wastewater change the geochemical properties of the subsurface environment over time.

Epidemiology Studies. The Health Effects Study investigated both short- and long-term health effects of reclaimed water, including assessing the possible health effects of reclaimed water using epidemiologic methods (Frerichs et al., 1981, 1982, 1983). The epidemiologic studies used two general approaches: geographic comparison or ecologic studies and a household survey.

In the ecologic studies, routinely collected data were used to calculate average rates of mortality and incidence in census tracts with "high" or "low" levels of reclaimed water. These rates were compared to rates in two control areas in which there had been no residential provision of reclaimed water. This type of comparison was made for numerous health outcomes for three time periods: 1969–1971, 1972–1978, and 1979–1980. The health outcomes included mortality (death from all causes, heart disease, stroke, all cancers, and cancers of the colon, stomach, bladder, and rectum), cancer incidence (all cancers, and cancers of the colon, stomach, bladder, and rectum), infant and neonatal mortality, low birth weight and congenital malformations, and selected infectious diseases (including hepatitis A and shigella). With few exceptions, there were only minor differences between the reclaimed water and control areas. The most noteworthy findings relate to higher standardized mortality ratios (SMRs) (or standardized proportionate mortality ratios, SPMRs) for rectal cancer in the reclaimed water census tracts. In the 1969–1971 period, the SMR was 1.67 (based on 18 deaths) in the "high" reclaimed water area and 1.17 (based on 45 deaths) in the "low" area. For the 1972–1978 period, the pattern was similar with a SPMR of 1.27 in the "high" area and 0.95 in the "low" area. In the 1979–1980 period, the SMR for rectal cancer *based on mortality data* was 1.52 (10 cases) for the "high" area and 0.63 in the "low" area (13 cases). For this same time period, 1979–1980, the SMR for rectal cancer *based on incidence data* was 0.82 for the high area and 0.60 for the low area, indicating no relationship with reclaimed water. Because cancer incidence data are considered to be more accurate and reliable than mortality data, it was concluded that the higher death rate due to rectal cancer did not accurately reflect the occurrence of the disease.

Another part of the epidemiologic study consisted of a telephone interview survey of adult females living in the "high" reclaimed water and control areas. The objective of this study was to investigate possible differences in spontaneous abortions and other adverse reproductive outcomes, bed-days, disability-days, perception of well-being, and health outcomes in an analysis that controlled for personal health status and consumption of tap water. This study concluded there were no significant differences in any of the health outcomes measured between women in the reclaimed water and control areas that could be attributed to differences in water quality.

Scientific Review of Health Effects Study

In 1986, the State of California appointed a Scientific Advisory Panel to review the status of information on health, technology, and monitoring aspects of recharging groundwater with reclaimed water (Robeck et al., 1987). As part of the review, the panel evaluated the design and methods used in the Health Effects Study. In its evaluation, the panel characterized the study as "thorough and well-conducted with state-of-the-art methodology." There were, however, concerns expressed regarding the limitations of the methods used in the Health Effects Study. The panel stated that the study showed that groundwater in the sampling sites is "contaminated with a variety of organic compounds of industrial, and perhaps treatment, origin," of which only about 10 percent were positively identified. Robeck et al. (1987) conclude that the data available from the characterization studies do not permit an unambiguous judgment regarding whether or not the majority of compounds present and of greatest health concern were identified. The panel also called for further work investigating the feasibility of a two-year oncogenicity protocol in rodents using water samples or water concentrates. The panel's final concern related to the epidemiologic studies' ability to detect an effect on human cancer. Panel members felt that the high population mobility in Los Angeles County and long latent period for human cancers (20 or 30 years or longer) could render the epidemiologic results related to cancer inconclusive.

Among the panel's recommendations were the following: (1) in any area, the highest-quality water available should be used for drinking, (2) the Whittier Narrows Groundwater Replenishment Project should continue, (3) surface spreading is preferable to injection as a means to recharge, (4) reclaimed water should be disinfected, but disinfection should not produce harmful by-products, (5) any new groundwater recharge project should conduct health surveillance of its population, (6) concentrates of reclaimed water should be tested for small amounts of harmful substances, (7) risk evaluation should be studied using animals in toxicology studies, and (8) monitoring for chemicals should be continued (Robeck et al., 1987).

UPDATE OF EPIDEMIOLOGIC ASSESSMENT

The present report provides information on rates of cancer, mortality, and infectious disease in an area receiving low levels of reclaimed water and a matched control area, both in Los Angeles County. Although the quality of reclaimed water is carefully monitored through extensive testing before and after recharge, epidemiologic studies differ from these types of analyses in two ways. First, studying the health of the population receiving reclaimed water enables us to observe the effects of past water quality even though historical information on the water quality is not available. Studies of water quality characterize samples at a single point in time or over a short period of time. These types of analyses cannot identify potentially harmful chemicals that may have been found in these water supplies months, years, or decades ago, or contaminants that may occur sporadically. Second, epidemiologic investigations are the only—albeit imperfect—way to study the effects on human health directly. Scientific studies in fields other than epidemiology focus on information that is only indirectly related to human health. Water quality studies are aimed at identifying individual chemicals, and toxicology studies are aimed at estimating the biological effect of each chemical. Neither water quality studies nor toxicology studies, however, can predict the synergistic interaction of these chemicals within the human system or their cumulative effect over years of chronic low-level exposure. Other types of scientific studies can add valuable information to an epidemiologic assessment, but cannot replace them (Ames, 1983).

This report provides a literature review, the detailed methods employed, and the results of the study. Chapter Two reviews the recent scientific literature on biologic, chemical, and radiologic contaminants of water, and epidemiologic studies of drinking water. Chapter Three describes the study methods: the assessment of the population's exposure to reclaimed water, the selection of control areas, the sources of data on health outcomes and population characteristics, and the statistical techniques employed in the data analysis. Chapter Four describes the characteristics of the populations living in the areas receiving reclaimed water and in the control areas. It also addresses the question of how the patterns of health outcomes compare in the reclaimed water and control areas, based on rates of cancer incidence, mortality, and infectious disease. Chapter Five discusses the study methods and results and the limitations of the study design.

Chapter Two

LITERATURE REVIEW

This chapter will acquaint the reader with the infectious agents and types of chemicals that may occur in drinking water, as well as with the results of epidemiologic studies of drinking water and health. Most of this review is not focused on reclaimed water, but rather on all types of potable water supplies.

The main challenge faced in maintaining any water supply for human consumption is to minimize the level of contaminants that may affect health. Determining what health effects are associated with potentially harmful constituents in drinking water is a difficult task. Such contaminants can be categorized as biological, chemical, and radioactive. The causal relationship between biological agents (protozoa, viruses, and bacteria) and disease has been well established. The effect of inorganic and organic chemicals on occurrence of disease in humans, however, is not well understood.

BIOLOGICAL CONTAMINANTS

Biological contaminants of drinking water have always been a concern to public health. Microorganisms indigenous to the aquatic environment are generally harmless, even in relatively high densities, for healthy human beings. Drinking water contaminated with human or animal fecal matter, however, may harbor bacteria, viruses, and protozoal organisms pathogenic to human beings (Craun, 1986). Historically, a major step in preventing waterborne outbreaks of diseases resulting from microorganisms was to isolate drinking water supplies from sewage disposal systems. By separating the two processes, the chain of transmission was interrupted. The practice of disinfecting water eliminated any microorganisms introduced into the water from other sources.

Today, standard disinfection procedures are being reviewed critically because experiments have shown that some viruses can survive secondary treatment and chlorination of sewage (Editorial, *British Medical Journal*, 1978). The effectiveness of chlorination depends upon temperature, pH, and the presence of organic matter, as well as the concentration and contact time with the disinfectant. Enteric viruses are much less sensitive to chlorine treatment than bacteria; they can survive in water for weeks and even months, and have a very low infective dose (i.e., even one virus particle can initiate an infection in a susceptible host) (Payment and Armon, 1989). Mechanical removal of viruses is in general considered ineffective because of the minute size of the virion (Robeck et al., 1987). Furthermore, viruses have been found in conventionally treated drinking water in the presence of residual chlorine (Payment, 1989). Payment and Armon (1989) reported that the efficiency of virus removal through wastewater treatment varies between 0 and 99.99 percent. The authors showed that for similar treatments, the effectiveness of virus removal differs greatly according to the type of virus, the type of treatment plant, and even the season of the year.

In the United States, the protozoal organisms giardia and cryptosporidium have raised recent concern. The oocysts of these organisms are resistant to chlorination and, therefore, water containing these oocysts should be treated by chlorination and filtration (Moore et al., 1992). Protozoal parasites other than giardia and cryptosporidium have created problems for recreational water use but not for drinking water safety during the last few decades (Moore et al., 1993; Levine et al., 1989; Herwald et al., 1991; Louis, 1986; Craun, 1986).

The Center for Disease Control, in collaboration with the U.S. Environmental Protection Agency, has maintained a surveillance program for waterborne disease outbreaks since 1971. Table 2.1 lists the organisms identified in all reported disease outbreaks resulting from water intended for drinking between 1985 and 1992 in the United States. The reporting of outbreaks is voluntary, however, and epidemics with milder symptoms might not be reported or might not be classified as an outbreak. Considering these limitations, this list of outbreaks probably represents only a fraction of actual outbreaks. Nevertheless, the summary suggests that most outbreaks— for public as well as nonpublic systems—and most cases in which an agent was identified were attributable to protozoal contamination with either giardia or cryptosporidium. In the acute gastrointestinal outbreaks for which no agent was identified, the symptom complex suggests a viral agent, which means viruses may be the second major cause of disease outbreaks from contaminated drinking water. In

Table 2.1

Disease Outbreaks Associated with Water Intended for Drinking, United States, 1985–1992

Infectious Agent	Public Systems		All Systems	
	Outbreaks (N=47) %	Cases (N=33,313) %	Outbreaks (N=128) %	Cases (N=49,300) %
Acute gastrointestinal disorder of unknown origin	27.7	35.6	54.7	39.2
Giardia lamblia	31.9	7.3	18.0	5.5
Cryptosporidium	6.4	48.0	3.1	33.6
Hepatitis A	2.1	<0.1	2.3	0.1
Norwalk virus	0.0	0.0	3.1	12.9
E. coli 0157:H7	2.1	0.7	0.8	0.5
Shigella	4.3	5.5	6.3	6.2
Salmonella	6.4	0.4	2.3	0.3
Camphylobacter	4.3	1.2	2.3	0.8
Cyanobacteria (algae)	2.1	0.1	0.8	<0.1
Chemicals	12.8	1.2	6.3	0.8

SOURCES: Louis (1986), Levine et al. (1989), Herwald et al. (1991), Moore et al. (1993).

about half of the outbreaks, a temporary interruption of disinfection, a chronically inadequate disinfection, or absent or inadequate filtration was listed as the probable cause of the system failure. With the exception of hepatitis and acute chemical poisoning, the illnesses resulting from these outbreaks had a gastrointestinal symptomatology.

A Swiss study reported that any level of classical fecal indicator bacteria above zero in drinking water was associated with an excess of acute gastrointestinal illness (Zmirou et al., 1987). Although fecal contamination of a drinking water source is confirmed by fecal coliform and enterobacteria growth, bacteria are unreliable indicators of viral or protozoal contamination. Moreover, no single organism has been found to date to correlate perfectly with the presence of human viruses in drinking water, indicating that there is no completely reliable indicator to substitute for viral analysis. Most enteric viruses are difficult to culture from water, but recent immunologic, molecular biologic, and genetic methods have permitted a more rapid and precise analysis of many human viruses. These methods, however, do not yield information regarding the viability of the organism. Thus, the results are equivocal with respect to human health significance.

The issue remains that not being able to identify one specific pathogen with a test does not mean many others are not in the same water sample. Most viruses detected in drinking water during the 1980s were enteroviruses (polio, coxsackie, and echoviruses), but reports of the presence of adenoviruses, reoviruses, and rotaviruses are becoming more frequent with improved detection methods (Payment and Armon, 1989). However, health effects have rarely been associated with the detection of these viruses. Payment and Armon (1989) argue that (1) health effects resulting from these viral agents might be less apparent or less recognized, (2) infections remain asymptomatic and thus are building immunity in the population, and (3) the effect attributed to waterborne sources might be small compared with other sources of infection. The authors' first argument is corroborated by the results of a randomized clinical trial in which the health effects of drinking domestically filtered tap water were compared with drinking unfiltered tap water (Payment et al., 1991). The authors estimated that about 35 percent of the gastrointestinal illnesses recorded in their study were attributable to the consumption of extensively treated river (i.e., surface) water meeting current microbiological drinking water standards. These intestinal illnesses were regarded as clinically significant infections, but as unlikely to have been recorded by a registry as waterborne disease outbreaks.

A major public health concern throughout the world is the rapid spread of the human immunodeficiency virus (HIV). There is no concern, however, about HIV being transmitted through water, for two reasons:

1. This virus could not be transmitted by water because of its instability and its sensitivity to heat, dessication, and commonly used disinfectants (Riggs, 1989; Gover, 1993). Unlike enteric viruses that replicate in the human intestinal tract and are shed in high numbers into domestic wastewater with feces, HIV cannot replicate in the intestinal tract and, therefore, is not present in feces. HIV can be introduced into domestic wastewater only via human blood or other bodily secretions.

Because these substances are much less likely to be introduced into the wastewater system than feces and at a much lower volume, only small numbers of HIV, if any, would be found in the receiving wastewater.

Researchers have added HIV to water experimentally to determine its ability to survive. Viable HIV were extracted from primary and secondary nonchlorinated effluents of conventional wastewater treatment plants. One study concluded that HIV is fairly stable in *nondisinfected* wastewater for up to 12 hours (Casson et al., 1992). Suspended solids and the organic load of wastewater seemed to enhance the survival of the virus in water. Another experiment showed that when the virus was added to dechlorinated tap water, no infectious viral activity was observed after 24 hours and the HIV lost 99.9 percent of its infectivity within 1 to 2 hours (Moore, 1993). These experiments support the hypothesis that HIV does not survive in routinely disinfected wastewater.

2. The second reason there is no concern about HIV being transmitted by municipal wastewater is the only way HIV can enter the body is through the bloodstream. The only recognized methods of transmission are (1) needles shared with HIV-infected intravenous drug users, (2) sexual intercourse with an HIV-infected person, (3) transfusion of blood or blood products containing HIV, (4) exposure of health-care workers to blood or body fluids from HIV-infected persons through an accidental needle stick or contact with an open wound, and (5) HIV-infected-mother-to-baby transmission in utero (Riggs, 1989). There have been no reports of HIV transmission by casual contact, soiled articles of any type, or any substance in the environment, including water.

For these two reasons, it can be concluded that HIV could not be transmitted through wastewater.

CHEMICAL CONTAMINANTS

Chemical components in the water are divided into two broad categories, inorganic and organic. Organic chemicals arise naturally in the water from decaying vegetation and animal tissue, animal excrement, photosynthetic by-products, and extracellular releases of organic matter by plankton and aquatic macrophytes. The type of inorganic constituents occurring naturally in water depends largely on the soil and geology with which the water comes into contact as well as the solubility of their inorganic components. Organic and inorganic contaminants of human origin enter water through domestic, agricultural and industrial wastes, accidental spillage, rainfall, seepage, non-point-source runoff, and improper land disposal of wastes.

Inorganic Chemicals

Several of the inorganic elements for which drinking water guidelines have been recommended by the World Health Organization (WHO, 1984) are recognized to be essential elements in human nutrition. Deficiencies in selenium and zinc have even been linked to increased cancer rates (Peeters, 1992). Nevertheless, excessive ingestion of these substances over time can be potentially harmful. The WHO (1984) considered 37 inorganic constituents of water, but decided to recommend guidelines related to potential health effects for only nine of them (Table 2.2). Table 2.3 lists the guidelines as well as those recommended by the State of California, the U.S. Environmental Protection Agency, and the WHO with regard to inorganic constituents of water.

Inorganic chemicals in wastewater that cause concern about human health include nitrates, sodium, heavy metals, and fluorides (Bruvold, 1981). The primary sources for undesirable inorganics are urban runoff and point sources for trace elements; agricultural sources, urban runoff and private waste disposals for phosphorus; and agricultural runoff for nitrogen and sediment (Moffa, 1983). Accidental contamination of drinking water with high levels of inorganics such as nitrate, chlorine, fluorine, and heavy metals has caused acute poisoning (Craun, 1986). A delayed problem arises from the ability of some inorganics to cause adverse health effects after accumulating in the body over prolonged periods of time. Heart disease and cancers have been associated in an epidemiologic study with chronic arsenic ingestion resulting from well water contamination (Wu et al., 1989). Nickel in drinking water has been suggested as a cause of bladder cancer (Peeters, 1992), and chronic low-level lead exposure—regardless of the exposure source—is known to impair children's IQ (Needleman et al., 1990). Cadmium reportedly increases the risk of prostate cancer, but only at relatively high concentrations found in occupational settings (Sullivan et al., 1988).

Organic Chemicals

Exposure to organic chemicals in drinking water is ubiquitous. Ram (1986) states that on a worldwide basis as of 1981, 2221 organic chemicals present at nanogram-to-microgram concentrations have been identified in water supplies, 765 of which were found in finished drinking water. Forty-three of these are suspected or positive carcinogens and 56 are known to be mutagens. More than 150 slightly-to-very toxic organic compounds were listed as having been found in tap water. Ram estimated that individuals using a single drinking water source would probably be exposed to less than 100 of these agents. Table 2.4 (Ram, 1986) gives an overview of the classes of organic compounds identified in water.

The first class of organic contaminants for which maximum contaminant levels (MCLs) were established was pesticides in public water supplies. The MCLs were set by the U.S. EPA National Interim Primary Drinking Water Regulations (December 1975) and the U.S. EPA Quality Criteria for Water recommended for the domestic water supply (1976). Pesticides are generally found in drinking water at levels far below permissible standards (Ram, 1986).

The chloroorganic compounds (e.g., trihalomethanes or THMs) that form during chlorine disinfection of water containing organic material have recently received considerable attention. These compounds have mutagenic and carcinogenic poten-

Table 2.2

Inorganic Constituents with Potential Health Significance

Constituent	Guideline Values Set	Background Document Drafted	Referred for Consideration of Aesthetic and Organoleptic Aspects	No Action Required
Aluminum			X	
Antimony				X
Arsenic	X	X		
Asbestos		X		
Barium		X		
Beryllium		X		
Boron				X
Cadmium	X	X		
Chromium	X	X		
Cobalt				X
Copper			X	
Cyanide	X	X		
Ferrocyanide				X
Fluoride	X	X		
Hardness (calcium and magnesium)		X	X	
Iron			X	
Lead	X	X		
Lithium				X
Magnesium			X	
Manganese			X	
Mercury	X	X		
Molybdenum				X
Nickel		X		
Nitrate	X	X		
Nitrite				X
Selenium	X	X		
Silver		X		
Sodium		X	X	
Tellurium				X
Thallium				X
Thiocyanate				X
Tin				X
Titanium				X
Tungsten				X
Uranium				X
Vanadium				X
Zinc			X	

SOURCE: *Guidelines for Drinking Water Quality*, Vol. 1, *Recommendations*, WHO, Geneva, 1984.

tial and occur universally in drinking water supplies (though in different concentrations), arising from the widespread practice of drinking-water chlorination. Whereas about 90 percent of the volatile organic compounds formed during the chlorination of water have been identified (and, because of their volatility, are relatively easily removed from water by aeration), only 35 percent by weight of all nonhumic, nonvolatile materials are known. However, nonvolatile chlorination by-products are associated with 98 percent of the mutagenic activity of chlorinated drinking water (Ram, 1986).

Table 2.3

Guidelines for Inorganic Chemicals in Water Intended for Drinking

Parameter	Drinking Water Standards[a] Primary (mg/L)	Secondary (mg/L)	EPA-MCLs[b] (mg/L)	WHO Guidelines[c] (mg/L)
Asbestos	7 MFL[d]	—	7[e]	—
Aluminum[f]	1.0	—	—	0.2
Antimony	0.006	—	0.006	—
Arsenic	0.05	—	0.05	0.05
Barium	1.0	—	2.0	—
Beryllium	0.004	—	0.004	—
Cadmium	0.005	—	0.01	0.005
Chromium	0.01	—	0.05	0.05
Chloride[f]	—	500	—	250
Copper[f]	1.3[g]	1.0	—	1.0
Cyanide	0.2	—	0.2	0.1
Fluoride	1.4–2.4	—	4	1.5
Iron[f]	—	0.3	—	0.3
Lead	0.015[g]	–	0.05	0.05
Manganese[f]	—	0.05	—	0.1
Mercury	0.002	—	0.002	0.001
Nickel	0.1	—	0.1	—
Nitrate + nitrite	10	—	10.0	10.0
Nitrate (as NO_3)	45	—	1.0[e]	—
Nitrite (as nitrogen)	1.0	—	—	—
Selenium	0.05	—	0.01	0.01
Silver	—	0.1	0.05	—
Sulfate[f]	—	500	500[e]	400
Thallium	0.002	—	0.002	—
Zinc[f]	—	5.0	—	5.0

[a]*California Safe Drinking Water Act and Related Laws*, 4th Edition, Title 22, Chapter 15, Articles 4 and 16, 1996.

[b]U.S. Environmental Protection Agency maximum contaminant levels (Lauer, 1993; Federal Register, July 17, 1992).

[c]World Health Organization (WHO), 1984.

[d]MFL = million fibers per liter.

[e]US-EPA proposed MCL.

[f]Aesthetic quality guidelines.

[g]Safe Drinking Water Act amendments, 1994.

RADIOLOGIC CONTAMINANTS

Radioisotopes or radionuclides can be classified as man-made or natural, and are further frequently categorized by their primary mode of decay emission (alpha, beta, and gamma). The natural radionuclides are largely alpha particle emitters with some beta particle activity from their progeny. The most significant natural radionuclides as determined by their levels of occurrence in drinking water and their potential to cause adverse health effects by this exposure route are radon-222, radium-226, radium-228, and uranium. Uranium minerals are found in the earth's crust in rocks and soil at different concentrations. Uranium-238 and radium-226, the parents of radon in the decay series of U-238, are relatively immobile, whereas radon is an inert gas that readily migrates from bedrock and soil into the groundwater or air.

Table 2.4

Classes of Organic Compounds Identified in Water

Naturally Occurring Compounds		
Alcohols	Carbohydrates	Nucleic acids
Aldehydes	Carboxylic acids	Organic acids
Aliphatic acids	Enzymes	Organophosphorus
Alkals	Esters	Peptides
Alkenes	Glucides	Protein
Amides	Heterocycles	Purines
Amino acids	Humic substances	Pyrimidines
Amines	Ketones	Steroids
Aromatic acids	Nitrogenous substances	Vitamins
Aryl alkanes	Nitrosamines	

Synthetic Compounds	
Aromatic compounds	Mercaptans
Bases, neutral organic compounds	Methane and ethane derivatives
Chemical brighteners	Neutral intractibles
Chlorinated acids	Nitro and nitroso compounds
Chlorinated aldehydes	Non-volatile acids
Chlorphenols	Organometallic compounds
Cyanides and azo compounds	Pesticides
Drug metabolites	Pharmaceuticals
Esters	Phenols
Ethers	Pigments
Extractable acids	Plasticizers
Food additives	Polynuclear aromatic compounds
Haloform	Quinones
Halogenated aliphatic compounds	Solvents
Halogenated aromatic compounds	Sulfated products
Halogenated carboxylic acids	Surfactants
Herbicides	Unsaturated hydrocarbons
Household chemicals	Volatile acids
Industrial chemicals	

SOURCE: Ram, 1986, p. 13.

Table 2.5 contains the maximum contaminant levels (MCLs) for radionuclides in drinking water proposed by the U.S. Environmental Protection Agency (Federal Register, 1991). A survey of drinking water wells throughout Southern California showed that 24 percent of all tested groundwater had levels of more than 500 pCi/L (PicoCuries per liter) and 62 percent had levels between 200 and 500 pCi/L for radon-222. If drinking water standards were set at less than 500 pCi/L for radon-222, 24 percent of groundwater supplies would have to be withdrawn from the water supply, or treated or diluted before distribution. Similarly, if drinking water standards were set at less than 200 pCi/L for radon-222, 86 percent of groundwater supplies would have to be withdrawn from the water supply, or treated or diluted before distribution (Black and Veatch, 1990). Because waterborne radon readily transfers to the air during normal use in the home, radon in water can contribute to the radon level in air and thus may increase the risk of lung cancer.

Man-made radionuclides enter the water through inadequate disposal of nuclear wastes and spills from nuclear facilities, chemical laboratories, and medical institu-

Table 2.5

**Proposed Maximum Contaminant Levels for Radionuclides
in Community and Nontransient, Noncommunity
Public Water Systems**

Radionuclide	MCL
Radium-226	20 pCi/L
Radium-228	20 pCi/L
Radon-222	300 pCi/L
Uranium	30 pCi/L
Beta and photon emitters (excluding Ra-228)	4 mrem ede/yr[a]
Adjusted gross alpha emitters (excluding Ra-228, U, and Rn-222)	15 pCi/L

SOURCE: Federal Register, Proposed Rules, Vol. 56, No. 138, July 18, 1991, 33051–33062.

[a]The unit mrem ede/yr refers to the dose ingested by a person drinking two liters of water per day over 50 years.

tions using radioactive materials. Radioactive materials could pose problems if drinking water were contaminated by any of these sources. Whereas many alpha emitters occur naturally (as described above), finding beta-emitting radionuclides with high toxicity in water should stimulate concern about discharges from nuclear operations into the water.

Bean et al. (1982) studied the health effects of radionuclides in water. This study compared the cancer incidence rates in 1969–1978 for Iowa residents whose drinking water came solely from wells over 500 feet in depth and not treated to remove radioactivity. The highest radioactivity group was defined as more than 5 pCi/L and the lowest as less than 2 pCi/L of mean radium-226 concentration measured over a 20-year period starting in 1958. Radium-226 was used as a marker for radionuclides in the water. Bladder and lung cancer incidence rates in both sexes and breast cancer in females increased with an increasing level of radium-226 in the water, but only the increase in male lung cancers was statistically significant. The ratio of rates among males—comparing the highest with the lowest exposure to radioactive water contaminants—was 1.7 for lung cancer and 1.4 for bladder cancer.

Bean et al. doubted that these results are attributable to smoking habits since they found a lower proportion of smokers in the municipalities with the highest radium-226 levels in the drinking water. A strength of the study lay in the restriction to deep wells as sources of drinking water, which avoided confounding with other chemical contaminants mainly found in surface and shallow well waters.

ECOLOGIC STUDY DESIGN

In an epidemiologic study with an ecologic design, the unit of analysis is a group of people, not an individual; information on exposure and disease outcome is available only at the group level. Expressed in more quantitative terms, the numbers of people with and without disease are known, and the numbers of people exposed and unexposed (i.e., the marginal distribution of these factors) are known. We do not know, however, whether the diseased individuals in our population are those who were exposed (i.e., the joint distribution of both factors)(Morgenstern, 1982).

The following discussion of the ecologic study design draws heavily from Greenland and Morgenstern (1989), Greenland (1992), and Walter (1991a,b). The loss of information in an ecologic study compared with an individual-level study gives rise to what is called the *ecologic fallacy* or *ecologic bias*. Because we do not have individual-level information, we have to assume that the observed intergroup variations reflect the valid relationship between disease and exposure at the individual level. An ecologically measured association can be either stronger or weaker than the same association evaluated at the individual level. In an ecologic study, in addition to concern about confounding (i.e., other risk factors for the disease that vary with the exposure) and effect modification (i.e., other risk factors that change the exposure effect) at the individual level, there must also be concern about confounding and effect modification at the group level.

We have to make two assumptions to conclude that no ecologic bias has occurred. First, we must assume that the groups are completely comparable with respect to every other possible risk factor for the disease to make sure that the background disease rates (in the absence of exposure) do not vary among the groups (i.e., no confounding by group). Second, we must assume that the exposure effect does not vary across groups (i.e., no effect modification by group). Risk factors that result in ecologic bias may not be confounders or effect modifiers at the individual level.

Without individual-level data, it is impossible to identify whether this type of bias exists in a study. Also, adding a variable to a multivariate model to control for confounding (such as a measure of socioeconomic status) can bias the ecologic effect estimate, instead of adjusting for confounding as would be expected on the individual level. When only ecologic data are available, the investigators must rely on prior knowledge of the characteristics of the groups being studied. They should attempt to match the control group to the exposed group as closely as possible with respect to factors that might affect rates of the disease being studied.

The recommended method for analyzing ecologic data is regression analysis. If ecologic subgroups are homogeneous with respect to exposure, regression will yield unbiased effect estimates. Thus, we are interested in defining subgroups in which exposure is distributed as homogeneously as possible. In the absence of confounding, an ecologic effect estimate is not distorted if each group is 100 percent exposed or a 100 percent unexposed. Multiple regression analysis, in which many possible confounding risk factors are included in the model, relies on many assumptions and can be easily misspecified. Furthermore, in an ecologic regression analysis, the problem of multicollinearity (where risk factors are mutually correlated) is much more pronounced than in individual-level studies, because the aggregated information ignores the exposure variation within groups.

EPIDEMIOLOGIC STUDIES OF DRINKING WATER

Studies of the health effects of reclaimed water fall into two categories: investigations of reclaimed water that has been *intentionally* reused and studies of reclaimed water that has been *unintentionally* reused. Although there are few studies of the health effects of "intentionally reused" reclaimed water, many studies of chlorinated surface water have been conducted in the last 15 years. The communities in these studies are usually downstream from industrial and municipal centers and receive chlorinated surface water—in other words, "unintentionally reused" reclaimed water. Thus, it seems reasonable to use investigations of chlorinated surface water as a guide to possible health outcomes in a study of the health effects of intentional reuse of reclaimed water.

Before reviewing these studies, the results of a few early studies of reuse of reclaimed water will be summarized. The results of the earlier epidemiologic studies of reclaimed water in the Montebello Forebay were summarized in Chapter One.

Studies of Reclaimed Water

One of three early studies concluded that consumption of reclaimed water caused acute illness. During droughts, reclaimed water was piped directly into the drinking water supplies of two communities, first in Iowa in 1940 (Brown, 1940) and again in Kansas in 1956–1957 (Metzler et al., 1958). The primary concern at the time was illness attributable to microorganisms, but no such effects were observed, perhaps because little effort was invested in finding such cases. A similar situation occurred in Germany in 1959, when river water was used for potable purposes (Zoeteman, 1977). The outcome of this episode, however, was different: A gastroenteritis of unknown origin was observed in some 7 percent of the population drinking the water.

Studies of Chlorinated Surface Water

Many studies of the possible effects on health of organic chemicals in drinking water rely on water source as an indicator of the level of organic chemicals in the water rather than of the specific compounds. Numerous early studies investigating the relationship between chlorination (or chloroform levels) and cancer found some correlation between cancer and residence in areas with chlorinated surface water (Wilkins et al., 1979). A New Orleans study reported a relationship between the percentage of Mississippi River water in drinking water and mortality rates from all cancers, urinary cancers, and gastrointestinal cancers (Page et al., 1976). The results of this study, however, were refuted on the basis of methodologic problems (DeRouen and Diem, 1975, 1977). Analyses of county-level cancer rates in Ohio led to the conclusion that counties with surface water supplies had higher rates of stomach cancer, bladder cancer, and all cancers combined (Kuzma et al., 1977). A study in New York state found no correlation between trihalomethane levels and cancer incidence rates (esophagus, stomach, colon, rectum, bladder, and pancreas) (Carlo and Mettlin, 1980). Another study in the state of New York reported a higher risk of gastrointestinal and urinary tract cancers among those with chlorinated water supplies (Alavanja et al., 1978).

More recently, Morris et al. (1992) conducted a meta-analysis of data related to the relationship between chlorination by-products in drinking water and cancer, based on results from nine case-control studies[1] and one cohort study[2] (Table 2.6). Based on this meta-analysis, the authors concluded that an association between bladder and rectum cancer and chlorination by-products exists. Furthermore, when the meta-analysis was restricted to studies with better measures of exposure, the overall relative risk for bladder and rectum cancer increased and the confidence interval narrowed. In addition, a dose-response relationship was observed when exposure was grouped into several categories. For all other cancer sites (i.e., brain, breast, colon, esophagus, kidney, pancreas, liver, and lung), the results from the studies varied and the quantitative meta-analysis showed no statistically significant association between chlorinated surface water and cancers of the various sites (Morris et al., 1992). However, the ability (power) to detect a relative risk of 1.2 (the same magnitude as the effect described for bladder cancer) was limited for cancer sites other than bladder and rectum (Table 2.6). Although the authors claimed to have conducted a meta-analysis of the carcinogenic effect of chlorination by-products, few geographic regions in the studies were supplied water from the same source in a chlorinated form to some consumers and nonchlorinated (mostly chloraminated) form to other consumers. A difference in chlorination practices almost always implies different water sources—chlorinated surface water versus nonchlorinated groundwater—and thus differences in possible chemical contamination of the drinking water sources.

This meta-analysis has been criticized for including case-control studies that analyzed death certificate data (Cantor, 1994). Because the data were derived from death certificates, many of the studies in the meta-analysis were not able to control for confounding variables. In addition, little or no historical information on drinking water quality was available in many of the studies. Finally, mortality data may be affected by the patient's access to care (i.e., those with better access may experience lower mortality). The case-control studies of chlorinated surface water and cancer based on death certificate data are summarized in Table 2.7. The case-control and cohort studies based on incident (new) cases of cancer are considered to be more re-

---

[1]Case-control studies are a type of epidemiologic study designed to evaluate the relationship between a specific exposure and some disease (Last, 1983). These studies start with identifying people with the disease of interest and an appropriate control group of people without the disease. The relationship between the exposure and the disease is studied by comparing how frequently the exposure is present in the two groups, diseased (case) and not diseased (control). This type of study is also known as a retrospective study.

[2]Cohort studies are another type of epidemiologic study designed to investigate the connection between an exposure and a disease (Last, 1983). These studies identify people who have been exposed and people who have not been exposed to a factor hypothesized to influence the probability of a disease occurring. The exposed and unexposed groups are observed for a number of years to generate reliable estimates of disease rates for the two groups. This type of study is also called a follow-up, longitudinal, or prospective study.

Table 2.6

**Results of Morris et al. (1992) Meta-Analysis on Selected Epidemiologic
Studies of Chlorinated Surface Water and Cancer**

Cancer Site	n[a]	Relative Risk Estimate	95 Percent Confidence Interval[b]	p[c]	Power[d] for Detection of Specified Relative Risks for $\alpha=0.05$[e]		
					1.20	1.40	1.60
Bladder	7	1.21	1.09, 1.34	<0.0001	—	—	—
Brain	2	1.29	0.53, 3.14	0.56	0.06	0.11	0.18
Breast	4	1.18	0.90, 1.54	0.24	0.27	0.69	0.93
Colon	7	1.11	0.91, 1.35	0.32	0.48	0.63	>0.99
Colorectal	8	1.15	0.97, 1.37	0.10	0.54	0.97	>0.99
Esophagus	5	1.11	0.85, 1.45	0.43	0.27	0.69	0.93
Kidney	4	1.16	0.89, 1.51	0.23	0.27	0.71	0.94
Liver	4	1.15	0.94, 1.40	0.16	0.44	0.92	>0.99
Lung	5	1.01	0.86, 1.18	0.94	0.27	0.69	0.93
Pancreas	6	1.05	0.91, 1.22	0.48	0.70	>0.99	>0.99
Rectum	6	1.38	1.01, 1.87	0.04	—	—	—
Stomach	6	1.14	0.94, 1.38	0.19	0.46	0.93	>0.99

[a]Number of studies evaluating specific cancer site.

[b]The numbers in this column represent the lower and upper limits of the 95 percent confidence interval around the relative risk estimate.

[c]The probability of the relative risk being equal to the number in the third column given the hypothesis that the relative risk is equal to 1.0.

[d]Statistical power is defined as the probability of detecting a difference when there is in fact a difference.

[e]The significance level or α (alpha) is the probability of finding a difference when in fact there is no difference.

liable indicators of an association, because incidence data are not subject to the same biases as mortality data. These studies are summarized in Table 2.8.

Three case-control studies were published after the Morris et al. (1992) meta-analysis was conducted. These studies are summarized at the bottom of Table 2.8. Two of the three studies corroborate the relationship between bladder cancer and chlorinated surface water consumption (Vena et al., 1993; McGeehin et al., 1993) and one study suggests an association with pancreatic cancer (IJsselmuiden et al., 1992). Interestingly, in McGeehin et al., 1993, the increased bladder cancer risk was associated only with chlorinated surface water whereas no effect for chlorinated groundwater was found. The authors thus suggest that chlorination might have been a surrogate for other chemicals contained in surface water.

The results of all published ecologic (i.e., geographic comparison) studies with respect to the cancer-causing potential of drinking water are summarized in Table 2.9. Most ecologic studies used county- or city-based mortality or incidence rates; only one study chose census tracts as a basis for analysis (Carlo and Mettlin, 1980). Thus, exposure homogeneity for the larger regions employed in the analysis is questionable

Table 2.7

Summary of Case-Control Studies of Chlorinated Surface Water and Cancer Based on Death Certificates

Authors	Outcome and Population	Exposure Assessment	Results
Zierler et al., 1986, 1988[a]	51,645 kidney, bladder, stomach, pancreas, colon, lung, breast cancer deaths. Controls: deaths from cardiovascular, cerebrovascular, pulmonary disease or lymphatic cancer by death certificate; Massachusetts residents	Chlorination at address on death certificate	Increased risk for bladder cancer, higher risk for lifetime exposure (>40 years) than for usual exposure (>21 years and <40 years)
Lawrence et al., 1984	395 colorectal cancer deaths vs. noncancer deaths matched 1:1 for age and sex by death certificate; New York female teachers	20-year employment and residential history with model for chloroform levels	No effect for female colorectal cancer
Gottlieb et al., 1982	10,205 kidney, bladder, stomach, liver, and colorectal cancer deaths. Controls: Two groups of cancer deaths and one of noncancer deaths, matched 1:1 for age, sex, race, and parish by death certificate; Louisiana residents	Chlorinated/unchlorinated water at address on death certificate and birthplace	Increased risk for female breast, and kidney and rectal cancer for both genders
Brenniman et al., 1980	3208 gastrointestinal and urinary tract cancer deaths vs. noncancer deaths matched 14:1 for age, sex, and county by death certificate; white residents of Illinois	Chlorinated/unchlorinated water at address on death certificate	Increased risk for colon and colorectal cancer
Young et al., 1981	8029 cancer deaths vs. noncancer deaths matched 1:1 for age, sex, race, and county by death certificate; white female residents of Wisconsin	Chlorinated/unchlorinated water at address on death certificate	Increased risk for female brain, breast, colon, and colorectal cancer

SOURCE: Part of the information in this table was taken from Tables 1 and 3 of Morris et al. (1992).

[a]The second study by Zierler (1988) was conducted on the same population as the 1986 study, but was limited to bladder cancer.

Table 2.8

Summary of Studies of Chlorinated Surface Water and Cancer Based on Incident Cases of Cancer

Authors	Outcome and Population	Exposure Assessment	Results
Cantor et al., 1987	2982 newly diagnosed cases of bladder cancer vs. community controls matched 2:1 for age, sex, and region by random dialing and Medicare files; white residents of 10 U.S. regions	History of residence and beverage consumption combined with survey and sampling of water utilities	Increased risk of bladder cancer
Young et al., 1987	347 newly diagnosed cases of colon cancer vs. general population controls matched 2:1 for age and sex; Wisconsin residents	Water consumption by interview and chloroform by historical records and measurement	No significantly increased risk for colorectal cancer
Cragle et al., 1985	200 newly diagnosed cases of colon cancer vs. noncancer hospital controls matched 2:1 for age, sex, vital status, and hospital; patients of 7 North Carolina hospitals	Years of exposure to chlorinated water by residential history and survey of water utilities	Decreased risk for colon cancer
Wilkins et al., 1981[a]	Diagnosis of cancer in 12 years following initial survey; 31,000 residents of Washington County, MD	Exposed: users of chlorinated surface water in Hagerstown, MD; Unexposed: deep well users	Increased risk for female breast cancer
Vena et al., 1993	351 newly diagnosed cases of bladder cancer compared to 855 community controls; white, male residents of western New York	Tap water consumption at the time of interview, most subjects used chlorinated surface water from the Great Lakes	Dose-response relationship between amount of tap water consumption and bladder cancer
McGeehin et al., 1993	327 bladder cancer cases matched to cancer cases other than colorectal or lung by sex and age, white population of Colorado	History of residency since age 20, drinking water source and recent beverage consumption combined with historical water quality information	Dose-response relationship for amount of tap water consumption and for duration of exposure to chlorinated surface water and bladder cancer. No significant trend for trihalomethane levels and bladder cancer
IJsselmuiden et al., 1992	101 pancreatic cancer cases, 206 controls, randomly sampled from 1975 census, Washington County, MD	Drinking water source municipal or nonmunicipal as ascertained in 1975 census	Increased risk of pancreatic cancer for municipal water consumers

SOURCE: Part of the information in this table was taken from Tables 1 and 3 of Morris et al. (1992).
[a]Wilkins et al. (1981) was a cohort study. All other studies in this table were case-control studies.

Table 2.9

Summary of Ecologic Studies of Chlorinated Surface Water and Cancer

Authors	Outcome and Population	Exposure Assessment	Results
Page et al., 1976	Mortality rates for total cancers, intestinal cancers between 1950–1969 for 64 Louisiana parishes	Proportion of parish population drinking water from the Mississippi River or its distributaries: 32% of the population living in the parishes in 1960 were supplied with river water, 56% with groundwater and 12% with other surface water. Of those supplied with Mississippi water, almost all received >60% of their water from this source	Mississippi water consumption increased total cancer mortality in white males, non-white males and females, urinary tract cancers in white males and non-white females, and gastrointestinal cancers in all groups
Kuzma et al., 1977	Average annual cancer mortality rate for whites by county as listed on death certificate as usual residence, 1950–1969 for 88 Ohio counties	Classification into groundwater users (42 counties) vs. surface water users (46 counties) based on water source provided to the majority of the county in 1960	Surface water use associated with increase of total cancers, stomach and bladder cancers in males and stomach cancer only in females. Restriction to counties with a more homogeneous exposure with respect to water source did not change the results
Cantor et al. 1978	Age-adjusted cancer mortality rates for whites in 1968–1971 in 76 U.S. regions studied in 1975 in which >65% of the population was served by a single water supply and >50% of the county was urban	THM and chloroform concentrations in the water supplies studied: THM levels ranged from .005–1 umol/L and chloroform levels from .003–4 umol/L	For all regions studied, bladder cancer in females was associated with increasing THM levels; this association was seen for men only in the northern regions
Hogan et al. 1979	Age-sex-adjusted cancer mortality rates for whites by county, 1950–1969 for about 156 U.S. counties	Organic contaminant levels in finished drinking water supplies of 163 water treatment facilities in 1975: chloroform levels ranged from .5–134 ug/L in 12 cities sampled twice	For counties in which >50% of the population had been served by water sources tested in the EPA surveys, chloroform levels were associated with large intestine and rectum cancer in males and large intestine and bladder cancer in females

Table 2.9—continued

Authors	Outcome and Population	Exposure Assessment	Results
Carlo et al., 1980	Registry-based age-adjusted cancer incidence rates, 1973–1976 for Erie County, NY	Census tract specific information on water quality, THM, chloroform, and pre-filtration chlorine levels and water source, surface vs. groundwater: 90% of census tracts were surface water users, 10% groundwater users, THM values had a range of 71 ppb	THM concentration associated with pancreatic cancer among white males only. "Surface" water source associated with esophageal and pancreatic cancers in the total population
Bean et al. 1982	Registry-based age-adjusted cancer incidence rates by municipalities based on address at time of diagnosis, 1969–1981 for Iowa towns with population size >1000	Classification of water source: surface (25 towns), shallow (57 towns), and groundwater users (39 towns had medium wells, 32 towns deep wells) for municipalities obtaining more than 90% of their drinking water from either water source between 1965–1979	Surface water use associated with increase in lung and rectum cancer in both males and females independent of municipality population size. Male and female rectal cancer rates decreased with increasing well depth
Beresford, 1983	Registry-based cancer incidence rates for 1968–1974 by borough restricted to age group 25–74 years for 14 London, UK boroughs	Proportion of river water ("reused" water) mixed with well water before distribution between 1926 and 1975: 6 boroughs classified as 1% reuse; 4 as up to 9% reuse; and 4 as up to 14% reuse (i.e., Thames River/well mixture)	Proportion of reuse associated with stomach, all urinary and bladder cancers in both sexes in unadjusted analysis. After adjustment for covariates only the results for females were marginally statistically significant
Isaacson et al., 1985	Registry-based age-adjusted cancer incidence rates by municipalities based on address at time of diagnosis, 1969–1981, for Iowa towns with population size >1000, groundwater users only	Measurement of volatile organic compounds and heavy metals in 1979; non-THM volatile organic compounds were detected in 5–55% and nickel in 20–40% of finished water supplies from ground sources	1,2-dichloroethane levels associated with male colon and rectal cancer regardless of chlorination status, female rectal cancer rates increased but not significant. Chlorinated groundwater sources associated with both cancer types. Nickel concentration associated with bladder and lung, as well as male colon and female rectal cancer
Morin et al., 1985	Total cancer mortality rates in 1949–50, 1959–1961, and 1969–1971 for 473 U.S. cities with population size >25,000 in 1950	Proportion of drinking water taken from surface water sources in the early 1950s	Increased total cancer mortality with increasing proportion of surface water use

Table 2.9—continued

Authors	Outcome and Population	Exposure Assessment	Results
Marienfeld et al., 1986	Age-adjusted cancer mortality rates for 1960–1967, 1972–1973 for St. Louis County and St. Louis City	Increase in THM and chloroform concentrations in St. Louis City due to a change in chlorination practice in 1955 of Missouri River water, which is the common drinking water in both areas	Relative increase of stomach, liver, large bowel, and bladder cancers as well as brain and cervix cancers from the period 1960–1967 to 1972–1976 in St. Louis County compared to St. Louis City
Wigle et al., 1986	Age-standardized mortality rates for the cities based on places of usual residence on death certificate, 1973–1979 for 66 Canadian cities with population size >10,000	Water source (i.e. surface, mixed, and groundwater), TOC, chlorine, THM, and chloroform concentrations	TOC (total organic carbon) concentration associated with cancers of the large intestines, including rectum in males only
Carpenter et al., 1986	Age-adjusted cancer mortality rates restricted to the age group 25–74 years for 253 urban areas in England, Wales, and Scotland	Water sources with respect to THM and chloroform concentrations in 1975; groundwater and natural springs classified as low, upland water medium for THM and high for chloroform, and lowland river water high for both.	Upland water associated with increase in female stomach and intestinal cancer
Griffith et al., 1989	Age-adjusted cancer mortality rates per county in 1970–1979, whites only, for 339 U.S. counties with hazardous waste sites compared to all other 2,726 U.S. counties	Groundwater source within 4.8 km from the hazardous waste site found by EPA to be chemically contaminated in 1984 laboratory analyses; analytic evidence for 198 chemical compounds from trichloroethylene to mineral spirits	Increased odds ratios for cancers of lung, bladder, stomach, large intestines, and rectum in men and women, also for esophagus and prostate in men and breast cancer in women. Regional subset analysis showed no clear overall pattern

unless the whole county or city was supplied with water from one common source. This was true only for the studies of drinking-water health effects in Iowa towns (Bean et al., 1982; Isaacson et al., 1985). Exposure assessment varied from classifying exposure according to water source to the measurement of specific chemicals, mostly trihalomethane, contained in the drinking water at certain points in time. In general, the ecologic study results support the results from the case-control and cohort studies: Bladder and rectum cancer rates increase with the extent of surface water use and the trihalomethane concentration in the drinking water. Drinking water contaminants were sporadically associated with various other cancer sites.

In summary, although many epidemiologic studies have investigated the relationship between drinking water and health, no consensus has been reached regarding the effects of drinking water containing low levels of chemicals. The literature suggests some water sources are associated with elevated risks of bladder and rectum cancer, but the evidence is far from conclusive.

Chapter Three

METHODS

Some reclaimed water has been used to recharge the groundwater basin for 30 years in the Montebello Forebay region of eastern Los Angeles County. During the 1960s, the domestic water supplies of this area contained a uniformly low percentage of re-claimed water. During the 1970s and 1980s, the percentage of reclaimed water re-mained low in some water systems, whereas other water systems experienced a gradual but steady increase in the percentage of reclaimed water, reaching a maxi-mum of 31 percent in some systems.

Using an ecologic study design, this epidemiologic study tested the hypothesis of an association between reclaimed water and a broad range of biologically plausible health outcomes. Existing data on cancer incidence (1987–1991 cancer registry records), mortality (1989–1991 death certificates), and infectious disease (1989–1990 reports to the health department) were analyzed in conjunction with population counts from the 1990 Census. Rates of the health outcomes were compared between an area in eastern Los Angeles County receiving some reclaimed water and a matched control area in Los Angeles County not receiving any reclaimed water. The census tracts receiving reclaimed water were allocated to five exposure categories based on the percentage of reclaimed water in their supplies. Poisson regression methods were used to compare disease rates in the reclaimed water and control areas.

SELECTION OF HEALTH OUTCOMES

A broad set of biologically plausible health outcomes was investigated in the study, because no specific cause-and-effect hypothesis related to reclaimed water has been developed. No biologic agents and only trace levels of a small number of chemical compounds have been found in groundwater replenished with reclaimed water in the Montebello Forebay (Nellor et al., 1984). We thus analyzed many different health outcomes, rather than limiting the study to a few health outcomes that are known to be or suspected of being affected by exposure to a specific chemical. The 28 out-comes analyzed include 9 related to cancer incidence, 13 related to mortality, and 6 related to infectious disease incidence.

The analyses of cancer incidence data address the important question of carcino-genicity. Eight specific cancer sites (Table 3.1) were selected based on associations found in previous studies of chlorinated surface water. (See Chapter Two for a discussion of these studies.) The cancer sites include the organs of the gastrointestinal and urinary tracts because of their exposure to ingested solids and liquids. Two cancer sites, bladder and rectum, have been associated consistently with chlorinated surface water and, therefore, were of primary interest in the analysis.[1] In addition, all cancer sites combined were analyzed to characterize the overall rate of cancer; the category of all cancers, however, was not hypothesized to be related to reclaimed water.

Mortality data were analyzed for 13 causes of death, including 9 cancer sites and 4 other causes (Table 3.1). The cancer categories were the same as for cancer incidence and were selected for the same reasons. In addition to cancer deaths, deaths due to all causes, diseases of the heart, cerebrovascular disease, and other causes were studied.[2] Mortality is considered to be a less-precise measure of an exposure effect than incidence and perhaps even biased.[3] These data, however, provide information on diseases not available from any other source (e.g., heart disease). In addition, these data allow comparisons to be made with the mortality results of the earlier epidemiologic studies of reclaimed water.

We analyzed data on six categories of infectious diseases (Table 3.1), based on the biologic agents implicated in recent waterborne outbreaks of illness in the United States and other countries (see Table 2.1). We were not able to analyze data on cryptosporidium, a protozoan that has been responsible for several waterborne outbreaks in recent years, most notably the 1993 outbreak in Milwaukee, Wisconsin (Blair, 1994). The Los Angeles County Department of Health Services did not collect information on cryptosporidium infections during this period.

EXPOSURE TO RECLAIMED WATER

An individual's exposure to chemical contaminants in the drinking water is deter-mined by two factors: the concentration of chemicals such as chlorination by-products and industrial pollutants in the tap water and the amount of tap water consumed. In determining how the timing of exposure might be related to disease incidence, the latent period between exposure and occurrence of the disease must also be considered. The crucial time of exposure to carcinogenic chemicals, however, is unknown. Therefore, ideally these factors would be evaluated over the

---

[1]The biological plausibility of this association being causal in nature is supported by the physiological function of these two organs. It has been suggested that the epithelial tissue of the bladder and rectum may be exposed to higher levels of ingested carcinogens because they store concentrated liquid and solid waste, respectively, prior to excretion (Morris et al., 1992).

[2]Even some of these other causes of death have been hypothesized to be related to water-quality characteristics. Water hardness has been hypothesized to be inversely related to cardiovascular disease. There is mixed evidence from studies designed to evaluate this hypothesis (Comstock, 1979).

[3]There are several reasons that mortality is considered to be a less precise measure of an exposure effect. First, not all cases of disease result in death. Using death rates, therefore, may underestimate the occurrence of the disease. Second, after people develop a disease, they may move to another location, making a geographic association between a disease (based on death information) and exposure difficult to establish. Third, people survive for different lengths of time after developing a disease, making a time association between death and exposure more difficult. Finally, some diseases are underestimated from death certificate information because they are not routinely listed on the death certificate as a cause of death.

Table 3.1

Health Outcomes Included in Analysis

Health Outcome	ICD-9 Code[a]
Cancer incidence	
All sites	140–208
Bladder	188
Colon	153
Esophagus	150
Kidney	189.0–189.1
Liver	155.0–155.2
Pancreas	157
Rectum	154.1
Stomach	151
Mortality	
All causes	—
Cancer	
All sites	140–208
Bladder	188
Colon	153
Esophagus	150
Kidney	189.0–189.1
Liver	155.0–155.2
Pancreas	157
Rectum	154.1
Stomach	151
Heart disease	390–398, 402, 404–429
Cerebrovascular disease	430–438
All other causes	—
Infectious disease	
Giardia	007.1
Hepatitis A	070.0–070.1
Salmonella	003
Shigella	004
Other	—
Amebiasis	006
Cholera	001
Gastroenteritis	009.2
Leptospirosis	100
Meningitis (not mumps)	322
Typhoid fever	002
All of the above	—

[a]Health outcomes of interest (cancer, death, and infectious disease) were identified in the data using International Classification of Disease, Ninth Revision (ICD-9) codes (International Classification of Diseases, 1994).

entire lifetime of a person, taking into account changes in residency, water sources, and water quality of each source. So far, no study of health effects related to drinking water has measured all of the factors for exposure assessment, and such a complete exposure analysis does not even seem feasible.

In this study, the residents of the reclaimed water and control areas were assumed to be exposed to the same amount of tap water over time. This implies that (1) they did not drink water from sources other than their home tap, or at least they drank the same amount from their home tap, and (2) they did not modify their tap water using domestic filters. In the absence of information on specific compounds, we have classified the water supplies dichotomously: (1) containing some reclaimed water and (2) containing no reclaimed water. The assumption behind this decision is that the chemical content varies more between sources than over time within the same source.

Although using the water source as a surrogate is the least-detailed measure of chemicals contained in the water, measuring individual chemical compounds in the water is not necessarily less prone to measurement error. Using a single measurement of one or very few substances to assess exposure forces the researcher to make some dubious assumptions: First, the chemicals measured are adequate markers for all other contaminants. Second, the measurement of the chemical(s) is reliable. Third, the measurements taken at one or two points in time reflect the historical chemical content of the water source accurately.[4] Some empirical data support the notion that single-year measurements are inadequate measures of exposure. Using information on source of water at one point in time as a surrogate for lifetime exposure to chemicals contained in a drinking water source has been found to have a fairly large effect on the results of epidemiologic studies.[5] In one ecologic study of drinking water and health, results changed depending upon the method used to classify the population according to exposure.[6]

Empirical estimates of the amount of tap water consumed by women living in the Montebello Forebay are available from a 1981 household survey (Frerichs et al., 1982). In this study, detailed questions about current consumption of tap water were asked of a sample of women 18 and older living in an area receiving reclaimed water and in a control area. Women living in census tracts within the reclaimed water area reported consuming 0.81 liters of tap water on a daily basis. Although this figure cannot be used to estimate reclaimed water exposure in the present study,[7] it indicates that a smaller volume of tap water is consumed in the reclaimed water area than in other areas where women reportedly consume 1.4 liters of tap water per day (Robeck et al., 1987).

---

[4]Hogan et al. (1986) reported wide variation in measured chloroform concentrations in the drinking water of 12 cities sampled and measured in two different surveys during the same year (e.g., a difference of up to 182 percent).

[5]Two study protocols allowed evaluation of this type of exposure misclassification bias in case-control or cohort studies. When Gottlieb et al. (1982) restricted their analysis to people whose lifetime source of drinking water was surface water or whose lifetime source was groundwater, the effect measures for cancer mortality increased compared with an analysis which used water source at the time of death only as a proxy measure for lifetime exposure. Lynch et al. (1989) compared four methods of estimating lifetime exposure within the same case-control study. They found that the more-detailed methods that included information on most or all drinking water sources from a lifetime residential history provided them with an exposure variable that was clearly showing a dose-response effect for water chlorination and bladder cancer.

[6]Cantor et al. (1978) showed results for subgroups of their study population with various degrees of exposure homogeneity. They found the highest correlations between chemical exposure in the drinking water source and bladder cancer when at least 85 percent of the population in a geographic area was served by the examined water source. The correlations disappeared when only 50–64 percent of the population was served by a drinking water source for which chemical contents had been analyzed.

[7]The control areas used in the 1981 epidemiologic study were different from those in the current study. In addition, to use information from a different time period and on different individuals might be only slightly better than using no information.

Estimating the Percentage of Reclaimed Water in Domestic Supplies

Estimating the percentage of reclaimed water in the water supplies of the Montebello Forebay was a critical first step in this research. Because reclaimed water cannot be labeled and traced through the system, the percentage of reclaimed water in household supplies must be estimated indirectly. The indirect estimation method was based on three empirical measurements: (1) the volume of reclaimed water used to recharge the groundwater basin, (2) the distance between the well(s) used by a water system and the point of recharge, and (3) the relative percentages of groundwater and surface water supplied to consumers by the water system. Each of these three factors was used in estimating the percentage of reclaimed water.

The volume of reclaimed water used to recharge the groundwater basin is the primary determinant of the percentage of reclaimed water in the groundwater pumped out of the Montebello Forebay of the Central Basin. Over the past 40 years, several sources of water have been used to recharge the groundwater basin, including imported surface supplies through the State Water Project Aqueduct conveying supplies from Northern California and the Colorado River Aqueduct providing water from the Colorado River, as well as storm runoff and reclaimed water. During the 1950s, the groundwater basin was recharged with water imported from the Colorado River and local storm runoff. In the early 1960s, groundwater recharge with reclaimed water began and recharge with other sources continued. In the mid-1970s, the volume of Colorado River water used for recharge diminished and was replaced with State Water Project supplies imported by The Metropolitan Water District of Southern California (MWD). The relative and absolute volumes of reclaimed water used to recharge the Montebello Forebay groundwater basin have increased over time. Therefore, it can be assumed that the proportion of reclaimed water delivered to consumers in the Montebello Forebay has also increased substantially.

The percentage of reclaimed water in a particular water supply in the Montebello Forebay also depends on the distance between the well(s) and the spreading grounds. In general, it takes less time for recharge water to reach wells located closer to the spreading grounds than wells that are farther away. The rate and direction of flow in the groundwater basin is also affected by factors other than distance, including basin geology, soil permeability, pumping rates, and basin hydraulic gradients (which reflect relative basin water levels). To account for this, the analysis incorporated data on the time it takes for water used for recharge to reach a well based on well water quality samples from locations throughout the basin, rather than only on the distance between the well and the spreading grounds.

The relative amounts of surface water and groundwater used by a single water system can fluctuate significantly from year to year and even from season to season within a single year. A mixture of groundwater and surface water supplies the residential, business, and industrial customers of water systems of the Montebello Forebay. Water systems personnel make decisions regarding the use of these two sources on the basis of availability and cost. Data on which water sources were used and how much of each source was used (production levels for individual wells) were incorporated into the estimates of the reclaimed water.

Estimating the percentage of reclaimed water supplied to residential customers in the Montebello Forebay was time-consuming. Data on the three factors discussed above—the volume of reclaimed water used in the recharge process, the replacement lag time for wells throughout the Montebello Forebay, and the relative amounts of groundwater and surface water used by each water system—were collected from regional water agencies and individual water systems. These data were then used in calculating the percentage of reclaimed water. The data collection and analysis were conducted by Bookman-Edmonston Engineering, Inc., an engineering firm specializing in water resources, and is documented in a separate report (Bookman-Edmonston Engineering, Inc., 1993a). In its report, Bookman-Edmonston Engineering, Inc. provides annual estimates of the percentage of reclaimed water for each water service area in the Montebello Forebay. The remainder of this section summarizes its methods and findings.

Identifying Water Purveyors in the Montebello Forebay

Most of the water systems operating in the Montebello Forebay area were included in our epidemiologic health effects study: 27 systems out of 39. The other 12 systems were excluded because the data needed to estimate the percentage of reclaimed water in their supplies were either unavailable or unreliable.[8] Subareas of four water systems were excluded because they served only nonresidential (i.e., business and industrial) customers.[9] See Table 3.2.

Several water systems in the Montebello Forebay contain more than one service area. Each service area was treated like a separate system in calculating the percentage of reclaimed water, because the operating parameters differ by service area, not by water system. There are 66 service areas contained within the 27 water systems included in the study.

Data on the operating practices of all water systems in the Montebello Forebay were collected by Bookman-Edmonston Engineering, Inc. for the 30-year period from 1960–1990. The information requested from each water system service area included the boundaries of its service areas, the number of residential connections, the sources of water used, and the production levels for each well within a service area. The staff at Bookman-Edmonston Engineering, Inc. used this information in determining the percentage of reclaimed water in the systems' supplies.

---

[8]Based on available information, the percentages of reclaimed water being served by these 11 water systems are probably less than 5 percent. Most of the excluded systems serve small populations located on the south and west edges of the Montebello Forebay.

[9]Another set of water systems was identified by Bookman-Edmonston as having received a small amount of reclaimed water at some time between 1977 and 1991. The amount of reclaimed water served by these systems, however, was too low to justify a complete analysis. Typically, these systems were located on the outer edges of the Montebello Forebay and had received less than 3 percent reclaimed water for a year or more. These areas were identified so they would not be considered as possible control areas.

Table 3.2

Montebello Forebay Water Systems Included and Excluded from Epidemiologic Assessment

Systems Included in Study	Map No.[a]	Systems Excluded from Study	Map No.[a]
Bellflower-Somerset Mutual Water	33	Bellflower Home Garden	36
California Water Service Company	1	Bigby Townsite	37
City of Downey	3	City of Commerce	5
City of Huntington Park	34	City of Compton	38
La Habra Heights County Water District	6	County Water Co.	39
City of Lynwood	24	La Hacienda Water Company	40
Maywood Mutual Water Company No. 3	25	Los Angeles County Water Works No. 10	41
City of Montebello	8	Lynwood Park Mutual Water Company	42
Montebello Land and Water Company	9	Maywood No. 1	43
Mutual Water Owners Assoc., Los Nietos	7	Maywood No. 2	44
City of Norwalk	10	Midland Park Water Trust	45
Orchard Dale County Water District	11	Park Water Company (part)	12J
City of Paramount	35	Peerless Land and Water Company (part)	26E,F
Park Water Company (part)	12	Walnut Park Mutual Water Company	46
Peerless Land and Water Company (part)	26		
Pico County Water District	13		
City of Pico Rivera	14		
Rancho Los Amigos	28		
San Gabriel Valley Water Company	15		
City of Santa Fe Springs	16		
City of South Gate	30		
South Montebello Irrigation District	17		
Southern California Water Company	18		
Southwest Suburban Water Company	19		
Tract No. 180 Mutual Water Company	31		
Tract No. 349 Mutual Water Company	32		
City of Whittier	20		

[a]Numbers refer to map of Montebello Forebay water system service areas (available upon request).

Estimating Percentage of Reclaimed Water in Groundwater Supplies

The first step in estimating the percentage of reclaimed water in household water supplies was to estimate the percentage of reclaimed water in the groundwater supply used by each water system service area. Groundwater in different parts of the Montebello Forebay of the Central Basin contains differing percentages of reclaimed water. Because reclaimed water cannot be measured directly, the percentage of reclaimed water in the groundwater supply was estimated indirectly using one or more of four statistical methods. Which technique to use depended upon what data were available for a particular service area. For some service areas, two or more techniques were used. For each service area, the percentage of reclaimed water in the groundwater supply was calculated for each year between 1960 and 1990.[10]

---

[10]Percentages for 1960-1976 were based on calculations performed as part of the Health Effects Study by the Los Angeles County Sanitation Districts and Bookman-Edmonston Engineering, Inc. (Nellor et al., 1984).

The four statistical techniques employed in the estimation process were (1) direct calculation from the sulfate ion model, (2) regression analysis, (3) the Kriging analytic method, and (4) an analysis of travel time contours.[11] Multiple methods were required because some techniques could not be used with the data available. In general, the sulfate ion model could be used as a "stand-alone" technique only for data from 1960 through 1982. Regression analysis was used for the subset of data between 1983 and 1990 with a correlation of 0.80 or greater between the results of this method and the sulfate ion model. The Kriging technique was used for 1983–1990 data with correlations lower than 0.80. The travel time contour method was used instead of the Kriging method for service areas in which no comparison wells were available. Using these four methods (described in Appendix A), Bookman-Edmonston Engineering, Inc. generated detailed data on the percentage of reclaimed water in the groundwater pumped by each water system service area in the Montebello Forebay.

Estimating Reclaimed Water Percentages by Service Area

The final step in estimating reclaimed water percentages incorporates information on how much groundwater is pumped by each water system. Water systems in the Montebello Forebay use a mixture of groundwater and surface water. Because only pumped groundwater (not surface water) contains reclaimed water, the percentage of reclaimed water served in any given year depends on the percentage of groundwater pumped by the water system during that year. For each water system, the average annual percentage of groundwater in the total volume of water served was estimated by the staff at Bookman Edmonston Engineering, Inc. using operations data obtained from the water systems. This information was used to calculate the annual percentage of reclaimed water in the total supply for each water system service area, as follows:

$$T_{rw} = T_{gw} \times G_{rw},$$

where T_{rw} =   percentage of reclaimed water in total supply

T_{gw} =   percentage of pumped groundwater in total supply

G_{rw} =   percentage of reclaimed water in pumped groundwater.

The percentage of reclaimed water in the total supply was calculated for each water year[12] between 1960 and 1990 for each of the 66 water system service areas. These percentages were used to classify the population into the exposure categories used in the analysis of the health outcomes data. (These data are reproduced in Appendix A.)

---

[11]Methods 2 through 4 were based on the sulfate ion model with the addition of other techniques to modify the results.

[12]A water year is the period October 1 through September 30.

Of the 66 service areas, 58 served some reclaimed water during the 30-year period; the remaining eight served no reclaimed water. The maximum annual percentage of reclaimed water in the water supplies served by the 58 water systems varied greatly. Fourteen service areas served an annual maximum of reclaimed water over the 30-year period between <1 and 4 percent, 19 served an annual maximum between 5 and 19 percent, and 25 served an annual maximum between 20 and 31 percent.

LINKING EXPOSURE DATA WITH OTHER DATA

Census tracts[13] were the unit of analysis in our study. We were able to link data on reclaimed water exposure with other data in the study at the census tract level. To do this, we compared the boundaries of the water system service areas and census tracts on a street map of the Montebello Forebay region. We identified 141 census tracts in the Montebello Forebay service areas that served reclaimed water sometime during the 30-year period. For many of these census tracts, the boundaries of the service areas and the census tracts did not match, and census tracts were split between two or more water systems. In those cases, the percentage of reclaimed water was calculated as a weighted average, with the weight based on the population in the census tract.[14]

A categorical variable representing exposure to reclaimed water was used in the statistical analysis instead of a continuous variable.[15] Each census tract was assigned to one of five exposure categories, based on its percentage of reclaimed water. The categories are labeled RW 1 (lowest level of reclaimed water) to RW 5 (highest level). The decision to use a categorical measure was based on exploratory analyses that indicated the relationship between the percentage of reclaimed water and disease rates was not linear. Transforming the reclaimed water percentage still did not produce a linear relationship. Under these conditions, use of a continuous exposure measure in the statistical analysis might yield a biased estimate of the effect of reclaimed water on disease rates.

---

[13]Census tracts are small geographically defined areas used by the U.S. Bureau of the Census to count the population of the United States every ten years. The average population size in a census tract is about 5000 people.

[14]For example, suppose two water systems (System 1 and System 2) served water in tract A. System 1 covers 20 percent of the population living in tract A and its water contains 10 percent reclaimed water. System 2 covers 80 percent of the population and its water contains 5 percent reclaimed water. A weighted average of the percentage of reclaimed water would be calculated for tract A as follows:

$$\text{Weighted average} = (0.20 \times 10\%) + (0.80 \times 5\%) = 6\% \, .$$

Therefore, in the analysis, tract A would be assigned to an exposure category based on the 6 percent. The assumption was made that the population was uniformly distributed within a census tract unless areas without housing were identifiable on the map (such as parks, colleges, and industrial areas).

[15]Using a categorical measure to estimate an exposure effect is not the most efficient method. Given our large sample size, however, a loss in efficiency was acceptable to avoid bias.

The use of exposure categories (rather than a continuous exposure measure) can also be justified given the quality of the exposure data. The percentage of reclaimed water is calculated from imprecise data and may be prone to measurement error for individual census tracts. We feel, however, that the majority of tracts have been accurately ordered by exposure level using the five categories. This approach has not completely removed the bias associated with measurement error, but it provides estimates of the exposure effect that can be justified given the quality of the exposure data.

For the cancer incidence and mortality data, the five categories of exposure were based on a 30-year average of reclaimed water percentages (Table 3.3). (See Appendix B for the census tracts in each category.) Exposures throughout the 30-year period might be important in determining the rate of cancer and death between 1987 and 1991. Many cancers are thought to have long induction periods, meaning that the period between exposure to a "cause" and the occurrence of disease may be decades. By analyzing cancers and deaths occurring in the late 1980s in relationship to an exposure that started in 1960, an implicit assumption is made that the latent period from exposure to disease is 30 years or less. Information about exposure to reclaimed water was used for the entire 30 years, rather than for only the first ten or twenty years because the role of causes in the carcinogenic process is unknown, and, therefore, the critical period for exposure is unknown. By using a 30-year average, information on exposure from the early years of the time period as well as from more recent years was incorporated. In addition, if we assume there is a threshold for the effect of reclaimed water (i.e., a percentage of reclaimed water above which an effect would be expected to occur), the higher percentages of reclaimed water in the 1980s may influence outcome rates more than the lower percentages in the 1960s and should be used to classify the census tracts. The rank order of the five exposure categories remained the same over almost the entire 30-year period (Figure 3.1).[16]

Table 3.3

**Definitions of Exposure Categories Used in Analysis of
Cancer Incidence and Mortality Data**

Exposure Category	Number of Census Tracts	Average % Reclaimed Water[a]	% Range of Reclaimed Water[b]
RW 1	41	0.3	0.0–0.9
RW 2	28	1.5	1.1–2.0
RW 3	30	3.0	2.1–5.0
RW 4	23	6.5	5.1–7.4
RW 5	19	11.4	9.0–15.2

[a]The average is calculated as a mean of all 30-year (1960–1990) averages for the census tracts in each exposure category.

[b]The range represents the minimum and maximum 30-year averages (1960–1990) among the census tracts in each exposure category.

---

[16]The only exceptions are RW 4 being higher than RW 5 in 1980 and RW 1 being higher than RW 4 in 1962.

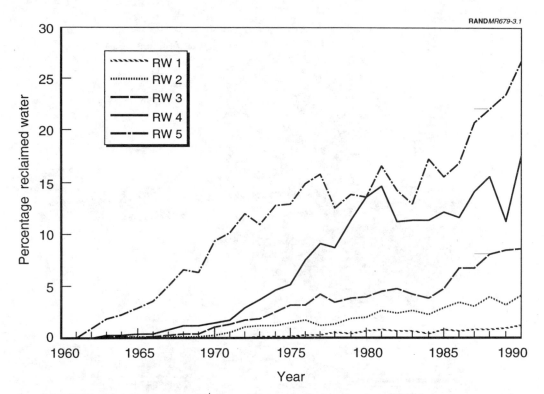

SOURCE: Based on data from Bookman-Edmonston Engineering, Inc. (1993a).

Figure 3.1—Percentage of Reclaimed Water by Year for Exposure Categories Used in Cancer and Mortality Analyses, 1960–1990

Thus, using exposure information from only the early years (e.g., before 1980) to allocate census tracts to exposure categories would have resulted in few differences from information on the entire 30 years.[17]

The census tracts receiving different levels of reclaimed water (RW 1 through RW 5) form a patchwork pattern in the Montebello Forebay area (Figure 3.2). In general, the areas with higher percentages of reclaimed water are located near the spreading grounds.[18] Because of a complicated distribution system and a large number of water systems, however, adjacent census tracts may be receiving markedly different percentages of reclaimed water.

For the infectious disease data, the five categories of exposure were based on a three-year average (1988–1990) of reclaimed water percentages (Table 3.4). (The census

---

[17]The Pearson correlation coefficient between the average exposure over 30 years (1960–1990) and the average exposure over the first 20 years (1960–1980) is 0.97.

[18]The spreading grounds are located next to the Rio Hondo on the border of Montebello (eastern side) and Pico Rivera (western side).

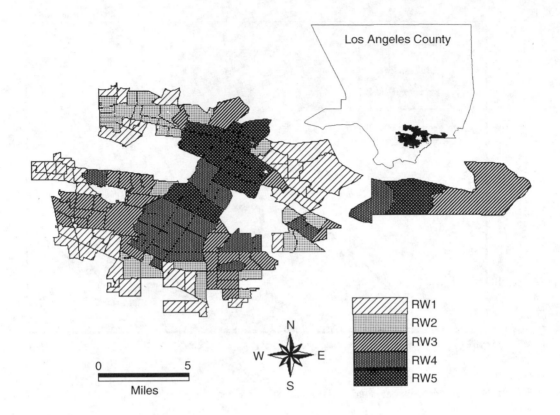

Figure 3.2—Map of Montebello Forebay Region of Los Angeles County: Census Tracts in Exposure Categories Used in Analysis of Cancer and Mortality Data

Table 3.4

Definitions of Exposure Categories Used in Analysis of Infectious Disease Data

Exposure Category	Number of Census Tracts	Average % Reclaimed Water[a]	% Range of Reclaimed Water[b]
RW 1	29	1.0	0.2–1.9
RW 2	27	3.1	2.0–4.9
RW 3	30	7.6	5.3–9.4
RW 4	25	13.7	10.6–17.9
RW 5	20	24.0	18.0–30.7

[a]The average is calculated as a mean of all three-year averages (1988–1990) for the census tracts in each exposure category.

[b]The range represents the minimum and maximum three-year averages (1988–1990) among the census tracts in each exposure category.

tracts in each category are listed in Appendix C.[19]) Because the incubation periods for most infectious diseases are days, weeks, or at most, months, only exposures near the time of the disease's occurrence could be related to the cause. These diseases would be expected to be diagnosed within a short time following exposure to the biological agent (protozoan, bacteria, or virus).

SELECTION OF THE CONTROL AREA

Selection of the control area was aimed at identifying an area in Los Angeles County that did not receive any reclaimed water, but otherwise had characteristics as similar as possible to the reclaimed water areas. Matching the characteristics of the populations living in the control area with those living in the exposed areas minimizes the effects of possible confounders[20] on the results. By matching the reclaimed water and control areas on confounding variables that may be important in determining disease rates, observed differences in outcomes will be more likely to be attributable to reclaimed water than to the other confounding variables. Matching the characteristics of the populations living in the control areas with those living in the reclaimed water areas has the added benefit of increasing the statistical power of the analysis (i.e., the probability that we will detect a difference when in fact there is a difference). Profiles for several possible control areas were developed, containing information on population characteristics as well as variables related to the relevant water supplies. The control area was selected from these candidates.

The control area was selected on the basis of characteristics as close as possible to the characteristics of the reclaimed water areas. In selecting the control area, we reviewed data on demographic and socioeconomic characteristics of the population (based on data from the 1990 U.S. Census), as well as information related to water sources and water quality provided by Bookman-Edmonston Engineering, Inc. The matching criteria included the following:

Characteristics related to sources of water:

- reclaimed water,

- groundwater contamination with volatile organic compounds (VOC);

Demographic characteristics of the population:

- size of population,

- percentage under 18 years of age,

- percentage 65 years and older,

- percentage Hispanic,

---

[19]Some census tracts that received reclaimed water in years preceding 1988 did not receive any reclaimed water between 1988 and 1990. These tracts were excluded from the analysis of infectious disease data.

[20]A confounder is a factor that is a determinant (or cause) of the outcome and is unequally distributed among those exposed and those not exposed. Not controlling for a confounder in an analysis results in "confounding," which is a distortion of a true effect of an exposure on an outcome by its association with other factors that can influence the outcome (Last, 1983).

- percentage of Spanish-speaking households,

- percentage non-Hispanic white,

- percentage non-Hispanic African-American,

- percentage non-Hispanic Asian;

Labor force characteristics of the population:

- percentage of employed persons in professional occupations,

- percentage of employed persons who are operatives, service workers, and laborers,

- percentage of labor force that is unemployed;

Income characteristics of the population:

- percentage of all families below poverty level,

- percentage of households receiving public assistance income in 1989;

Characteristics of the population related to citizenship:

- percentage of persons who are not U.S. citizens,

- percentage of persons under 18 who are not U.S. citizens,

- percentage of persons 18 and over who are not U.S. citizens,

- percentage who are foreign born;

Characteristics of the population related to education:

- percentage with less than or equal to 8 years of education,

- percentage with high school education,

- percentage with a bachelor's degree or more;

Characteristics of the population related to housing:

- percentage of housing units that are renter-occupied,

- percentage whose householder moved in during 1989–1990,

- percentage of population living in same house as in 1985.

Many areas in Los Angeles County were considered as a control for the Montebello Forebay region. Among the areas considered, several were found to differ in terms of demographic and socioeconomic characteristics from the Montebello Forebay. On this basis, the following areas were deemed inappropriate and eliminated from consideration:

- Artesia
- Lakewood
- Northern Long Beach
- Carson
- Gardena
- Lawndale
- West Covina
- Diamond Bar
- Torrance
- San Dimas
- Hawthorne

Other areas similar to the reclaimed water areas in terms of their demographic and socioeconomic characteristics had widespread VOC contamination of their groundwater supply. It was found in the mid-1980s that almost the entire San Gabriel Valley had widespread VOC contamination of the groundwater supply.[21] Areas eliminated from consideration because of groundwater contamination included

- cities located in the San Gabriel Valley

- La Puente

- The Eagle Rock, Glassell Park, Highland Park, and Mount Washington regions within the City of Los Angeles.

After an extensive search, we identified three locations in Los Angeles County to use as a control area matched with the areas receiving reclaimed water. These locations were chosen on the basis of demographic and socioeconomic characteristics similar to the Montebello Forebay, no known VOC groundwater contamination, and receiving no reclaimed water. The census tracts in the control area are widely dispersed throughout Los Angeles County: they are located in the Montebello Forebay (but receive no reclaimed water), in the Pomona area to the east, and in the northeastern San Fernando Valley to the northwest (Figure 3.3).

The first control location consists of the population living in 15 census tracts throughout the Montebello Forebay region. This area receives water from the eight water system service areas in the Montebello Forebay that have never served any reclaimed water to their customers, either because the pumped groundwater contains no reclaimed water or because the water system serves only surface water (not groundwater).

The second control location, Pomona, contains 21 census tracts in the eastern area of Los Angeles County. It was selected on the basis of the similarity of its residents to the population living in the Montebello Forebay. After the area was matched on the basis of population characteristics, the staff at Bookman-Edmonston Engineering, Inc. evaluated information from the City of Pomona on historical water quality in the Pomona area (Morgan, 1994a). The water served to Pomona residents is derived from three sources: groundwater wells, sources imported from outside the Los Angeles area by The Metropolitan Water District of Southern California, and surface supplies obtained from San Antonio Canyon. Pomona water supplies have never contained any reclaimed water.

The third and largest control location is the northeastern San Fernando Valley in northern Los Angeles County. It was selected on the basis of population characteristics similar to those of the Montebello Forebay. Of the 81 census tracts in the northeastern San Fernando Valley location, 78 receive surface water only from the City of Los Angeles Department of Water and Power. The remaining three tracts are supplied by the City of San Fernando water system, with a mixture of groundwater and

---

[21]The control area in the previous epidemiologic studies was located in the San Gabriel Valley (Frerichs, 1981, 1982, 1983).

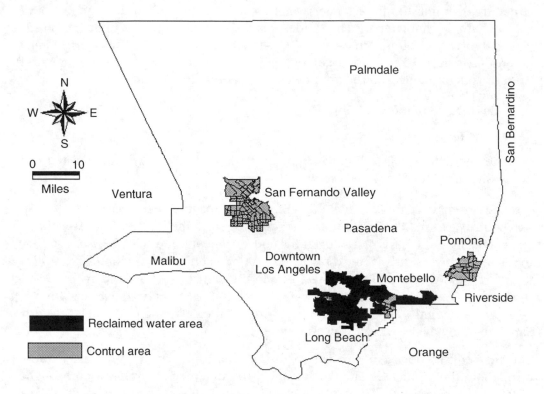

Figure 3.3—Map of Los Angeles County Showing Reclaimed Water and Control Areas

surface water. These supplies have never contained reclaimed water and have never been affected by groundwater contamination (Morgan, 1994b, 1994c).

DATA SOURCES

Information on health outcomes (cancers, deaths, and infectious diseases) came from existing data that are collected on a routine and ongoing basis by health agencies in Los Angeles County. There is reason to believe that few errors are made in the data collection process and, even more important, the error rate should not differ between the areas receiving reclaimed water and the control area. Thus, the quality of the data is probably uniform across all study areas.

Cancer Incidence

We analyzed all incident (new) cases of cancer occurring among residents of the reclaimed water and control areas for the five-year period from 1987 through 1991. The cancer data were obtained from the University of Southern California Cancer Surveillance Program (CSP). The computer files from the CSP contained the number of cancer cases for age, ethnicity, and gender-specific subgroups in every census tract in Los Angeles County by year of occurrence. The analysis covered nine categories of cancer: all cancers and eight specific types (see Table 3.1).

The CSP is a population-based cancer registry covering all of Los Angeles County. Cancer case reports are submitted to the CSP by all hospitals in the county. In addition, CSP technicians review all pathology reports at all hospitals and pathology laboratories at which cancer diagnoses are made. If a pathology report is found for which a hospital report has not been received, the hospital or physician of record is contacted and instructed to complete a report. A collaboration of ten regional registries conduct cancer registration for the entire state of California. If a Los Angeles County resident is diagnosed anywhere in the state, the local regional registry forwards the report to the CSP. Furthermore, all death certificates for Los Angeles County residents are screened by the CSP for any mention of cancer. For any death for which a report has not been received, the CSP contacts the hospital or physician of record to obtain a report. Thus, cancer reporting for Los Angeles County is assumed to be virtually complete.

Mortality

All deaths of residents of the census tracts in the reclaimed water and control areas during the three-year period from 1989 through 1991 were included in the analysis of mortality data. The data were obtained from the Los Angeles County Department of Health Services (DHS). The mortality information comes from death certificates recorded for every death as part of the registration system for vital events. Each death record was assigned a 1990 census tract at the DHS by an automated geocoding system based on the residential address at the time of death. The census tract allows the mortality data to be linked with the exposure and population data.[22] The analysis focused on 13 mortality categories: deaths due to all causes and 12 specific causes of death (see Table 3.1).

Infectious Diseases

Data on infectious diseases for residents of the reclaimed water and control areas were obtained from the Los Angeles County Department of Health Services. These data represent cases of notifiable diseases occurring in 1989 and 1990 that were reported to the DHS. They are known as "confidential morbidity reports." The analysis was restricted to several diseases that have been linked to waterborne outbreaks of illness in the United States or other countries (see Table 3.1). Each infectious disease record was coded with the 1990 census tract based on the residential address at the time of diagnosis, allowing linkage between the infectious disease records and the data on population and exposure.

Ascertaining the true incidence of infectious diseases is affected by several reporting-related problems. Some cases with milder symptoms might not be reported because they are not treated by a health care professional. In addition, reporting notifiable diseases by health care professionals is voluntary, increasing the chance of under-

---

[22]On the computer file received from the LACDHS, most of the 1989–1991 death records contained a variable indicating the 1990 census tract of residence. For the small proportion that were missing this information, RAND staff used the 1980 census tract variable to assign the 1990 census tract.

reporting. Further, some cases may be misdiagnosed or might not be reported for other reasons. Considering these limitations, the data on infectious diseases that appear in this report probably represent some fraction of the cases that actually occurred. There is no reason to believe, however, that there are differential rates of reporting in the reclaimed water and control areas (i.e., the proportion of cases reported in the reclaimed water areas differed from the proportion in the control areas). A comparison of rates in the two areas is probably not affected by under-reporting, and, therefore, is relatively unbiased.

Population

Data on the number and characteristics of persons living in the reclaimed water and control areas were derived from the 1990 Census of Population and Housing machine-readable files for California (Census of Population and Housing, 1991a, 1991b, 1991c). The count of persons by age and sex was derived from data from the Summary Tape File 1 (Census of Population and Housing, 1991a). The count of persons by age, sex, and race/ethnicity was derived from data from the Summary Tape File 2 (Census of Population and Housing, 1991b). The socioeconomic characteristics used to select the control areas and to describe the population living in the reclaimed water and control areas were calculated on the basis of data from the Summary Tape File 3 (Census of Population and Housing, 1991c).

Exposure to Water Contaminants Unrelated to Reclaimed Water

Identifying sources of possible groundwater contamination *unrelated to reclaimed water* was the final step in characterizing the study areas. Groundwater contamination can be caused by illegal dumping of chemicals, leaking underground storage tanks, or hazardous waste sites, all of which are unrelated to reclaimed water. If the water in the reclaimed water areas or in the control areas was affected by this type of groundwater contamination, it could confound the relationship between health outcomes and reclaimed water. Several sources were investigated to collect information on VOC groundwater contamination, radon, leaking underground storage tanks, and potentially leaking toxic waste sites in the region.

Volatile Organic Compounds. Volatile organic compounds are one of the most common groundwater contaminants and have been associated with various cancers and birth defects (Geschwind et al., 1992; Swan et al., 1992; Wrensch et al., 1985; Isaacson et al., 1985; Carlo et al., 1980; Wilkins et al., 1979; Zierler et al., 1988; McGeehin et al., 1993 IJsselmuiden et al., 1992; Vena et al., 1993). The federal government enacted regulations as the health risks became more widely understood and the routine monitoring for these contaminants in drinking water became commonplace by the mid-1980s.

A complete list of the first and highest incidence of VOC contamination for wells serving the Montebello Forebay was supplied by Bookman-Edmonston Engineering, Inc. Routine monitoring and analysis showed that 32 of the 159 wells in the Montebello Forebay had evidence of VOC contamination at or above the federal drinking water standards at least once between 1984 (when testing was first required) and 1991. According to follow-up interviews with the water purveyors conducted by Bookman-Edmonston Engineering, Inc., however, contaminated water was never served to the public. Water from these wells was either blended with other water or the well was shut down until contamination levels met federal standards. No records are available for this period, so these statements are based primarily on statements from personnel currently employed by the purveyors.

Similar information on VOC contamination was collected by Bookman-Edmonston Engineering, Inc. for the control area. Some groundwater contamination with VOCs has been detected in the Pomona water supply, but the levels were below the maximum contaminant levels (MCLs) and, therefore, considered safe for drinking according to federal regulations. Data on VOCs in the San Fernando Valley were available from the major domestic water purveyor, the City of Los Angeles Department of Water and Power (DWP), except for a small portion of the San Fernando Valley served by the City of San Fernando. Information supplied by DWP to Bookman-Edmonston Engineering, Inc. indicates that residents of the San Fernando Valley control area never received water above the MCL for VOCs since the testing program began in 1984.

Radon. Exposure to radon in air is considered to be a risk factor for lung cancer. Because radon in water can readily transfer to the air during normal water use in the home, radon in water may also increase the risk of adverse health outcomes. Currently, no maximum contaminant levels exist for radon in water, but the Safe Drinking Water Act requires the Environmental Protection Agency to establish MCLs for four radionuclides of greatest concern —radium-226, radium-228, natural uranium, and radon-222 (radon). The current proposed standard is 300 pCi/L (picoCuries per liter).

In 1990, The Metropolitan Water District of Southern California measured radon levels in 12 groundwater basins located in its service area to determine the impact various possible radon standards would have on its water supplies. The radon concentrations from 203 sampling sites varied between 93 and 1538 pCi/L, with an overall geometric average of 335 pCi/L (with 86 percent of the samples exceeding 200 pCi/L) (Black and Veatch, 1990). Radon levels for the region that included the Montebello Forebay ranged from 200 to 500 pCi/L. Levels for the control region of Pomona were also between 200 and 500 pCi/L, while the San Fernando Valley control region ranged from <200 to <1,000 pCi/L.

Information on radon levels was not available at the census tract level, and therefore could not be used in the analysis of health outcomes. It is unlikely, however, that radon in water would be a risk factor for the cancers analyzed in this study.

Leaking Underground Storage Tanks. The status of leaking underground storage tanks (LUSTs) in the Montebello Forebay was investigated by Bookman-Edmonston Engineering, Inc. (1993b) to determine the location of the tanks, impact on groundwater supplies, and remedial actions for those tanks containing hazardous substances. The firm concluded that 11 LUSTs might be affecting the groundwater of the Montebello Forebay by releasing solvents, heavy metals, or other trace organic compounds. The areas with possible contamination of the groundwater by LUSTs include the eastern edge of the City of Santa Fe Springs and the area west of the Rio Hondo in the cities of Montebello, Commerce, and Bell Gardens. The Pomona control area has only one leaking underground storage tank that might be affecting the groundwater supply.[23] With the exception of the City of San Fernando, the water supplied to the northeastern San Fernando Valley control area is surface water only and, therefore, is not affected by local groundwater contamination.

Several of the Montebello Forebay areas with LUSTs, including the City of Commerce and parts of Santa Fe Springs, were excluded from the study because they were industrial areas, not because of groundwater contamination. Four census tracts with LUSTs remain in the area because they were not found to differ in a way that would affect the conclusions of the study.[24]

Hazardous Waste Sites. Waste sites located in, or in close proximity to, the Montebello Forebay were investigated as possible sources of water contamination. We were concerned that these waste sites might be leaking hazardous substances into the groundwater basins. Bookman-Edmonston Engineering, Inc. reviewed the records of the State Department of Toxic Substances Control, the Environmental Protection Agency, and the Regional Water Quality Control Board for information related to waste sites. Based on this review, six hazardous waste sites were identified as potentially affecting the groundwater of this region with solvents, heavy metals, or other trace organic compounds (Bookman-Edmonston Engineering, Inc., 1993c). Four of the six sites—in the City of Santa Fe Springs and the City of Commerce—were considered major threats to the groundwater. Census tracts located near the six hazardous waste sites in the Montebello Forebay were not included in the analysis of health outcomes because the water systems and areas are used only for industrial purposes.

Control regions were evaluated for the presence of inactive hazardous waste disposal sites that might contaminate the groundwater supply; none were found. Two such sites have been identified in Pomona since 1984 (ABEX and Pomona Defense Supply Procurement Office). These sites have some soil contamination but no documented groundwater contamination (Personal communication, Miguel Monroy, Site Mitigation Unit, Department of Toxic Substances Control, Cal-EPA, March 1995). With the exception of a small area served by the City of San Fernando, the northeastern San Fernando Valley uses no groundwater; its drinking water supply, therefore, could not be adversely affected by any hazardous waste sites. For the small area served by the City of San Fernando, on only one occasion was the VOC contaminant perchloroethylene (PCE) detected at a low level. This small area of the San Fernando Valley served with groundwater supplies is not considered to be subject to contamination by a hazardous waste disposal site.

---

[23]The LUST in Pomona was identified on the Xerox site in Pomona in 1984, when the regulations went into effect. The site was found to contain solvents. According to the Los Angeles Regional Quality Control Board, any drinking water wells adjacent to the LUST were sealed immediately upon discovery of the contamination (Personal communication, Jose Pereyra, March 1995).

[24]The four census tracts are 5023, 5024, and 5320 in RW 5 and 5340 in RW 2.

STATISTICAL METHODS

The relationship between reclaimed water and disease and death rates was analyzed using multivariate regression techniques. All of the analyses control for the size of the population, age, and sex because these factors have the largest effect on the frequency of health outcomes. The number of events (health outcomes) occurring in a population depends primarily on the size of the population (i.e., more events would be expected in a larger population). After the first year of life, mortality increases steadily with increasing age. A population with more older people would be expected to have a higher death rate even with lower exposures to harmful substances. Controlling for age, therefore, is important in making a valid comparison between mortality rates in two populations with different age distributions. Similar increases in cancer incidence are observed with increasing age, whereas the incidence of infectious disease decreases with age. Males and females also exhibit different rates of cancer, mortality, and infectious disease, so controlling for sex is also necessary for a valid comparison.

The principal analyses control for ethnicity in addition to age, sex, and population size. Similar to the reasons above, we controlled for ethnicity because different ethnic groups experience different disease rates even in the absence of other differences. The results presented in the tables throughout Chapter Four are based on regression models that control for age, sex, ethnicity, and population size.

Regression Analysis of Health Outcome Data

We modeled the rate of disease or death as a function of demographic variables and exposure. For each census tract in our reclaimed water and control areas, we identified the number of cases of disease (or number of deaths) and the number of people in each age, ethnicity, and gender-specific subgroup. We then fit a model to the rate—number of cases (deaths) divided by number of people at risk—that assumes that for any given population count, the expected rate of disease depends multiplicatively on age, ethnicity, gender, and the exposure level for the census tract. A multiplicative relationship means that, for example, the rate of disease for women is always a fraction of the rate for men. In other words, the ratio of the rate for men to the rate for women is a fixed constant. Expressed in another way, this model states that the logarithm of the expected rate is an additive model with factors identifying age, ethnicity, gender, and exposure. Our model is

$$\log(R_{arse}) = \mu + \alpha_a + \beta_r + \gamma_s + \delta_e,$$

where R_{arse} denotes the expected rate of disease or death for people in the ath age group, of ethnicity r, of sex s, and in the eth exposure category. The parameters μ, α_a, β_r, γ_s, and δ_e are unknown and were estimated from our data (see Table 3.5 for the age, ethnicity, sex, and exposure categories used in the model). The parameter μ corresponds to the overall mean rate of disease (or death) across all groups and the individual group parameters denote deviations in the group mean from the overall

Table 3.5

Independent Variables Used in Regression Analysis

Characteristic	Definition of Regression Variable	Variable Name
Age (for cancer incidence)	Under 35 years	age00_34
	35 to 44 years	age35_44
	45 to 54 years	age45_54
	55 to 64 years	age55_64
	65 to 74 years	age65_74
	75 and older	*
Age (for mortality)	Under 45 years	age00_44
	45 to 54 years	age45_54
	55 to 64 years	age55_64
	65 to 74 years	age65_74
	75 to 84 years	age75_84
	85 and older	*
Age (for infectious disease)	Under 5 years	*
	5 to 14 years	age05_14
	15 to 24 years	age15_24
	25 to 64 years	age25_64
	65 and older	age65_99
Sex	Female	*
	Male	male
Ethnicity[a]	Hispanic	*
	Non-Hispanic white	white
	Non-Hispanic black	black
	Non-Hispanic other	other
Income[b]	Log(median family income)	lmedianf
Exposure to reclaimed water	Category 1 (lowest %)	expose_1
	Category 2	expose_2
	Category 3	expose_3
	Category 4	expose_4
	Category 5 (highest %)	expose_5
	Control	*

NOTE: * is the "omitted variable," a statistical term used in regression; it does not mean that this category was excluded from the analysis.

[a]Ethnicity was not used in the first alternative model in the sensitivity analyses.

[b]Income was used only in the second alternative model in the sensitivity analyses.

mean. For example, δ_1 would denote the rate difference between the rate for the lowest exposure category and the mean for the entire population.

To estimate the parameters of this model—the effects of age, sex, ethnicity, and exposure—we fit the model using maximum likelihood methods. We assumed that the number of cases of disease (the dependent variable) followed a Poisson distribution with a mean based on the disease rate and the population count. Maximum-likelihood estimates are the coefficient values that give the observed counts the highest probability they could have under the assumed model. If our assumed model is a reasonable approximation to the process generating the data, maximum-likelihood estimates have certain desirable statistical properties.

The parameter estimates generated by our Poisson regression model approximate the log of the ratio of the rate of disease (or death) in the exposed areas to the rate in the control area. We exponentiated these parameter estimates to generate the actual rate ratios (presented in Chapter Four). To create confidence intervals for the rate ratios, we calculated a 95 percent confidence interval for the parameter estimate and then exponentiated the upper and lower limits. The confidence intervals for the estimated coefficients were set at $s \pm 1.96 \times$ (standard error of s) where s is the estimate of δ. Because the estimated coefficients are approximately normal, this procedure produces a 95 percent confidence interval for the log rate ratio and the exponentiated interval yields a 95 percent confidence interval for the rate ratio.

The statistical significance of the effects in our models were tested using Wald tests. These tests are analogous to t-tests in regression modeling. Wald tests compare the test statistic to a chi-square distribution with the appropriate degrees of freedom.

Sensitivity Analysis

To test the sensitivity of the estimated exposure effects to the model parameters, we repeated the analyses of the health outcomes data with two alternative models. The first alternative model controlled for age and sex only, not for ethnicity. The second alternative model controlled for median family income (based on the 1990 U.S. Census) as an indicator of socioeconomic status, in addition to age, sex, and ethnicity.

The first alternative model analyses were conducted to observe the effect of removing ethnicity from the model on the estimates of exposure effects. Although we feel the "best" model would control for ethnicity, there was some concern that the definition of ethnicity, Hispanic in particular, may be different in the numerator and denominator. Different methods—which may not be comparable—are used to identify Hispanic individuals in the health outcomes data (numerator) and in the population data (denominator).[25] These differences may result in the same person being classified as Hispanic in the numerator and non-Hispanic in the denominator, a misclassification that might bias the results. The results from the model controlling for age, sex, and population size for cancer, mortality, and infectious disease are presented in Appendices G, H, and I, respectively.

The second alternative model controls for age, sex, ethnicity, population size, and—as an indicator of socioeconomic status—median family income. Because some

---

[25]For the cancer incidence records, a person is identified as Hispanic by the field representative collecting the data from the medical record or death certificate based on surname and other information available about the patient or decedent. For the death records, a decedent is identified as Hispanic by the next of kin, coroner, or presiding physician. For infectious disease records, a person is identified as Hispanic by the physician or public health agency filing the confidential morbidity report. Ethnicity is based on self-identification in the population data. Each person filling out a census questionnaire specifies the race and ethnic background (including Hispanicity) of each person in the household.

population characteristics differ between the reclaimed water and control areas, including income in the model tested the effect of controlling for differences in income on the estimates of exposure effects. The results from these models are also presented in Appendices G, H, and I.

Overdispersion

Models based on the Poisson distribution assume that the mean and the variance of the number of events (cases of disease or deaths) will be equal. Hence, the sub-groups (age, ethnicity, gender, and exposure groups) with a higher expected number of events should have a larger variance than subgroups with a lower expected number of events. Furthermore, the difference in the means should explain the difference in the variances. There are many reasons, however, why we might believe that the variance in the observed data will not actually equal the mean. We were concerned that we were not controlling for one or more variables that could cause the number of events to differ by tract and thus lead to greater variation than would be expected. This situation of larger-than-expected variance is known as over-dispersion. Because we have multiple cells (age by gender by ethnicity) for each tract, tract-to-tract differences could also lead to correlation among the deviations from the mean.

Both overdispersion and correlation can lead to underestimating the variability of our estimates and overstating statistical significance of differences between the reclaimed water and control areas. To account for deviations from the Poisson model, we used modified estimates of the variance suggested by Liang and Zeger (1986). This estimate does not rely on the strict assumptions of the Poisson model and allows for both correlation and overdispersion. All our statistical tests were conducted using these "robust" standard errors. These tend to be more conservative than tests made under the Poisson model, but they should prevent us from incorrectly identifying spurious differences among tracts.

Selecting Age Classes for Model Use

Age was the most important predictor of disease and death in the regression models. Initially, we tested 10-year age categories. To reduce the degrees of freedom in the model, we then collapsed age categories, retaining only those that represented different levels of risk. We also collapsed age categories to eliminate zero counts of disease or deaths. For example, the incidence of most cancers is very low among young people, so people under 35 years of age were grouped together for the study of cancer deaths. The selection of age classes was important for identifying age effects, but had little influence on our estimates of exposure effects. This results from the balanced nature of our design (same age groups in all tracts) and from the relatively homogeneous age distributions across exposure groups.

Inconsistency Between Numerator and Denominator

A few deaths and cases of disease occurred in age, ethnicity, and sex-specific sub-groups that had zero population. There are two possible explanations for this. First, because the cases and population were counted at two different times, the individual might not have lived in that census tract at the time of (or might have died before) the census enumeration. Second, ethnicity was identified differently in the health outcomes data and in the census data. This could lead to a situation, for example, in which the same person might have been identified as Hispanic in one system and as non-Hispanic white in the other. Because we could not estimate the rate of disease for cells with zero population, we could not include these cells in our analysis. This occurred infrequently, so excluding these cells should have little or no effect on the model.

Chapter Four

RESULTS

Rates of health outcomes were compared between two areas of Los Angeles County, one receiving some reclaimed water and the other receiving no reclaimed water. The health outcomes included cancer incidence (total cancers, and cancer of the bladder, colon, esophagus, kidney, liver, pancreas, rectum, and stomach), mortality (deaths due to all causes, heart disease, stroke, all cancer, and the eight specific cancer sites), and infectious diseases (giardia, hepatitis A, salmonella, shigella, and several less-common diseases). With few exceptions, the results indicate that cancer rates between 1987 and 1991, mortality rates between 1989 and 1991, and rates of selected infectious diseases in 1989 and 1990 were similar in the reclaimed water and control areas. The pattern of results is not consistent with a dose-response relationship between reclaimed water and the rate of disease. This epidemiologic study does not provide evidence that reclaimed water at the levels used in the Montebello Forebay has influenced the rates of cancer, mortality, or infectious disease. The observational nature of the study, however, makes conclusions regarding an effect or lack of an effect difficult.

CHARACTERISTICS OF STUDY AREA POPULATIONS

Study Areas in 1990

A total of 908,221 people live in Montebello Forebay census tracts receiving some reclaimed water in their water supplies, representing more than 10 percent of the population of Los Angeles County (Table 4.1). According to the 1990 U.S. Census, over 65 percent of the population receiving reclaimed water is Hispanic, with smaller percentages of non-Hispanic whites, blacks, and Asians. Almost one-third of those living in the reclaimed water area are not U.S. citizens, more than Los Angeles County as a whole. Compared to all of Los Angeles County, the reclaimed water area has a higher percentage of families below poverty level, a lower percentage of professional workers, and a much lower percentage of adults with education of a high school diploma or more. About half of residents of reclaimed water areas have lived in their residence for five years or more.

As described in Chapter Three, three locations were chosen to serve as a control area in the study: parts of the Montebello Forebay, the Pomona area, and the northeastern San Fernando Valley. The combined population of the three control locations

Table 4.1

Characteristics of Populations Living in the Reclaimed Water and Control Areas,
Based on the 1990 U.S. Census

Characteristic (in 1990)	Reclaimed Water Area	Control Area	Los Angeles County
Population	908,221	674,071	8,863,164
	Percent		
Hispanic	65.4	52.3	37.3
Non-Hispanic			
White	25.3	33.9	41.0
Black	3.2	6.0	10.7
Asian	5.4	7.2	10.4
Persons 0–17 years	31.3	29.6	26.2
Persons 65 years and older	8.8	7.8	9.7
Persons who are not U.S. citizens	28.6	29.7	23.7
Families below poverty level	12.6	11.7	11.6
Employed in white-collar occupations	16.3	19.7	27.6
Adults with eight years of education or less	25.3	21.3	15.6
Adults with high school education or more	54.6	61.0	70.0
Housing units that are renter-occupied	50.1	47.1	51.8
Living in same house for at least 5 years	51.0	44.9	47.2
Moved into current residence in 1989–1990	22.1	25.0	24.1

was 674,071, about three-quarters the size of the population receiving reclaimed water. Together, the reclaimed water and control areas contain almost 18 percent of the people living in Los Angeles County. The control area was matched as closely as possible to the reclaimed water areas. As a result, most demographic and socioeconomic characteristics are similar. Compared to the reclaimed water area, however, the population in the control area is somewhat less Hispanic (52 percent versus 65 percent) with more non-Hispanic whites, blacks, and Asians. In addition, the control areas have relatively fewer people who are not U.S. citizens, about the same percentage of families below poverty level, and more white-collar workers and adults with a high school education or more. About half of the residents of the control area had lived in the same house for five years or longer.

The population characteristics of the five exposure categories are shown in Appendix E for the cancer/mortality and infectious disease analyses. The five areas range in size from 116,000 people (RW 5) to more than 260,000 (RW 1). All areas are highly Hispanic, but RW 4 has a somewhat lower percentage of Hispanics. RW 4 and RW 5 appear to differ from the other three areas in several ways: a higher proportion of older people, fewer noncitizens, fewer families living in poverty, more professional workers, and fewer renters.

Increase in Size of Population Receiving Reclaimed Water, 1980–1990

The number of people receiving some reclaimed water in Los Angeles County increased from 478,182 in 1980 to 908,221 in 1990, almost a two-fold increase. The main reason for this increase is that by 1990, a larger geographic area was being served some reclaimed water. Between 1980 and 1990, reclaimed water migrated within the groundwater basin to points further away from the spreading grounds. The water pumped from wells in these more distant locations contained no reclaimed water in 1980, but by 1990 contained a low percentage. This resulted in a major expansion of the area and population receiving reclaimed water between 1980 and 1990. Increased density of the population (number of persons per household and number of households) may also have increased the population being served reclaimed water, although to a much lesser degree than the movement of reclaimed water in the groundwater basin. The data required to compare the population density at the two points in time are not available for analysis.

PATTERNS OF HEALTH OUTCOMES IN STUDY AREAS

Hypotheses Tested

Using an ecologic study design, we tested the hypotheses that rates of certain health outcomes are the same in areas with relatively low levels of reclaimed water and similar areas not receiving any reclaimed water. Our analyses are aimed specifically at comparing rates of cancer incidence, death, and selected infectious diseases using existing data. We selected the control area on the basis of population characteristics similar to the reclaimed water areas, in order to minimize the differences between the two areas that might affect the rates of cancer, death, or disease. For each health outcome, we compared each of the five reclaimed water areas with the control area. The five areas (RW 1, RW 2, RW 3, RW 4, and RW 5) are defined on the basis of increasingly higher percentages of reclaimed water.[1]

Sensitivity Analyses

Sensitivity analyses were conducted to assess the effect of different variables in the regression model on the results.[2] The results presented in tables throughout this chapter are based on a model that controls for the demographic characteristics that are most likely to affect the disease rates: age, sex, and ethnicity. Two alternative models were tested: one controlling for age and sex only, and the other controlling for age, sex, ethnicity, and family income. All three models control for population size. The results based on the alternative models are in Appendices G, H, and I, for cancer incidence, mortality, and infectious diseases, respectively.

Measures of Exposure Effect and Statistical Significance

For each health outcome, a rate ratio and a confidence interval around the rate ratio were calculated using the parameter estimates generated by the Poisson regression

---

[1]The five categories are defined in Chapter Three. For analyses of cancer incidence and mortality, census tracts were allocated to the exposure categories based on the average percentage of reclaimed water over the 30-year period (1960–1990), whereas the exposure categories for the infectious disease analyses were based on the percentage of reclaimed water over a three-year period (1988–1990).

[2]The rationale behind the three models is discussed in Chapter Three.

model. The rate ratio is a measure of effect commonly used in epidemiology. In this study, the rate ratio is calculated as the ratio of the rate in one of the reclaimed water areas (the numerator of the ratio) to the rate in the control area (the denominator of the ratio). A rate ratio greater than 1.0 indicates the rate is higher in the reclaimed water area than in the control area. A rate ratio less than 1.0 indicates the rate is lower in the reclaimed water area than in the control area. The estimated rate ratios are used to evaluate whether the rates in the five reclaimed water areas differ from the rate in the control area.

The upper and lower bounds of the 95 percent confidence interval represent a range of possible values for the rate ratio given the uncertainties associated with the data.[3] There is a direct relationship between the confidence interval and so-called "statistical significance." If the 95 percent confidence interval does not include the value of 1.0, the difference between the reclaimed water and control areas could be labeled as statistically significant (with a p-value of 0.05). The confidence interval should not be used only to reach a conclusion regarding whether the difference between two numbers is statistically significant (i.e., labeling a result as "statistically significant" or "not statistically significant"). The confidence interval also provides information on the uncertainty associated with the estimate as well as the size of the effect.

The results of all statistical comparisons conducted in the study are presented in this report. Another approach would be to present only those results that are statistically significant. The former approach is highly recommended by Thomas et al. (1985). In our comparisons, a fixed alpha level[4] of 0.05 has been assumed for all statistical tests. The number of statistically significant tests expected to occur by chance alone can be obtained by multiplying the alpha level by the total number of tests (Thomas et al., 1985).

Statistical significance is a tool that allows us to judge how probable or improbable a particular result is, but it does not reveal anything about the issue of cause and effect. Using statistical significance as the only criterion to decide whether a result is important may focus attention on the wrong subset of results. Some small (and perhaps meaningless) differences may be statistically significant because they are based on large sample sizes, whereas some large (and perhaps meaningful) differences may not be statistically significant because they are based on small sample sizes. Because statistical significance is highly dependent upon sample size, other criteria should also be considered in evaluating whether an association between an exposure and a health outcome is causal.

---

[3]A "95 percent confidence interval around the rate ratio" can be interpreted as follows. If a study based on this type of data was repeated in a similar population, the confidence intervals based on 95 percent of the replications would include the "true value" of the rate ratio, given the variability in the data.

[4]The alpha level or Type I error is the probability of finding a difference when in fact there is no difference. The level of acceptance of Type I error in a test of statistical significance is called the alpha.

Assessing Causality of Associations

If an association between reclaimed water and a health outcome is found in an epidemiologic study, it is important to consider whether the association occurred randomly or may indicate a causal relationship. In attempting to distinguish between causal and noncausal associations, several aspects of the association should be considered. Among these are strength, consistency, temporality, biologic gradient, plausibility, and coherence (Rothman, 1986; Hill, 1965).

The "strength" of an association refers to the magnitude of the rate ratio. In this study, rate ratios greater than 2.0 would be considered more indicative of a causal association between reclaimed water and a health outcome than rate ratios between 1.0 and 2.0, although the latter may also be of interest. "Consistency" of an association refers to the recurrence of the same finding under different circumstances (i.e., in studies of different populations at different times). If a relationship between reclaimed water and a health outcome were causal, results from studies conducted in different geographic areas or during different periods of time would be expected to yield the same result. "Temporality" of an association means that the cause must come before the effect. In the case of reclaimed water in the Montebello Forebay, if reclaimed water affects health, the effect would be expected to occur sometime after 1962 when groundwater recharge with reclaimed water began. The "biologic gradient" refers to a relationship between the cause and effect that follows a dose-response curve, with a larger effect (or response) occurring as a result of a larger exposure (or dose). If reclaimed water causes a health effect, disease rates would be expected to be higher in an area with more reclaimed water than in an area with less reclaimed water. "Plausibility" of the association refers to the biological basis for an association between a particular cause and an effect. In the case of reclaimed water, plausibility is difficult to demonstrate because no cause (i.e., a "potentially harmful" substance in reclaimed water) has been identified. If an increased rate of lung cancer were to be found in the areas with reclaimed water, however, it would be highly implausible that reclaimed water caused the lung cancer to occur given what is known about the biology of lung cancer. "Coherence" of an association refers to how well the scientific evidence supports an association between a cause and effect. This is similar to the plausibility criterion, but refers to the fact that interpreting an association as a cause and effect phenomenon should not conflict with accepted facts about the natural history and biology of the disease (Rothman, 1986). Each of these criteria should be addressed in evaluating the causal nature of an association.

The dose-response criterion is of particular interest when studying the health effects of reclaimed water. The wide range of exposure to reclaimed water in the populations being studied (from a minimum of 0 to a maximum of 31 percent reclaimed water in the water supplies) allows evaluation of a dose-response curve. If reclaimed water were causing a health effect, a dose-response relationship would be expected, with higher rate ratios in areas having higher percentages of reclaimed water.

NUMERICAL RESULTS

Cancer Incidence

For cancer incidence over a five-year period (1987–1991), rate ratios and confidence intervals were calculated for all cancers combined and cancer at eight specific sites (Table 4.2). These measures are based on newly identified cancer cases in the years under study. The number of cancers by cancer site can be found in Table F.1 for the five reclaimed water areas and the control area (Appendix F).

All cancers (i.e., cancer at all sites) occurred at about the same rate in the five reclaimed water areas and the control area. The two areas with the least reclaimed water (RW 1 and RW 2) had higher rates than the control area (1.06 and 1.13, respectively). Although the differences between the areas with the lowest percentages of reclaimed water and the control area are statistically significant, these differences are small in magnitude. Generally, the overall rate of developing cancer was about the same in all five areas receiving reclaimed water and in the control area.

The rates of bladder cancer and colon cancer are similar in the reclaimed water and control areas, based on rate ratios that are close to 1.0. The rate ratios in the five reclaimed water areas range from 0.85 to 1.03 for bladder cancer, and from 1.03 to 1.11 for colon cancer. The confidence intervals (CI) all include 1.0, meaning the rates in the reclaimed water areas are not statistically significantly different from the

Table 4.2

Rate Ratios and Confidence Intervals for Cancer Incidence, Controlling for Age, Sex, and Ethnicity, 1987–1991

Cancer site	Area					
	RW 1	RW 2	RW 3	RW 4	RW 5	Control
All sites	1.06[a]	1.13[a]	1.04	0.98	1.03	1.00
	(1.01–1.12)	(1.05–1.21)	(0.97–1.13)	(0.92–1.05)	(0.95–1.11)	
Bladder	0.95	1.01	0.95	0.85	1.03	1.00
	(0.77–1.17)	(0.80–1.29)	(0.80–1.13)	(0.68–1.06)	(0.80–1.32)	
Colon	1.09	1.08	1.04	1.11	1.03	1.00
	(0.95–1.25)	(0.93–1.24)	(0.92–1.19)	(0.94–1.32)	(0.89–1.18)	
Esophagus	1.23	1.27	1.17	1.20	1.29	1.00
	(0.80–1.87)	(0.78–2.06)	(0.64–2.16)	(0.85–1.69)	(0.73–2.28)	
Kidney	0.84	1.09	1.02	0.87	1.04	1.00
	(0.59–1.19)	(0.79–1.51)	(0.78–1.34)	(0.63–1.19)	(0.73–1.47)	
Liver	1.00	1.37	0.88	1.06	1.73[a]	1.00
	(0.62–1.61)	(0.87–2.17)	(0.54–1.42)	(0.73–1.55)	(1.10–2.74)	
Pancreas	1.09	1.11	1.25	0.88	1.05	1.00
	(0.86–1.39)	(0.82–1.50)	(0.96–1.62)	(0.68–1.13)	(0.75–1.48)	
Rectum	1.09	0.89	1.09	1.09	0.97	1.00
	(0.84–1.40)	(0.65–1.21)	(0.86–1.37)	(0.84–1.42)	(0.69–1.37)	
Stomach	1.08	1.29[a]	1.12	0.99	0.85	1.00
	(0.85–1.38)	(1.02–1.64)	(0.91–1.38)	(0.79–1.24)	(0.65–1.12)	

[a]95 percent confidence interval does not include 1.0, which would indicate a statistically significant finding (p < 0.05).

control areas. In addition, the rate ratios (RR) do not increase with increasing percentages of reclaimed water.

The rate ratios for esophagus cancer are slightly higher than 1.0 in all five of the reclaimed water areas. The confidence intervals are wide, however, with the lower limits below 1.0 and the upper limits above 1.0, indicating no meaningful differences between the reclaimed water areas and the control area. In addition, a dose-response relationship is not indicated by the fairly uniform magnitudes of the rate ratios in the five areas, all within the range of 1.17 to 1.29, with the lowest in RW 3 and the highest in RW 5.

No association between kidney cancer and reclaimed water was evident from analysis of the incidence data. Rate ratios in the five reclaimed water areas are slightly above and below 1.0 (ranging from 0.84 to 1.09), indicating the rates are close to the rate in the control area. The pattern of the rate ratios in the five areas does not indicate a dose-response relationship.

The rate of liver cancer in RW 5, the area with the highest percentage of reclaimed water, is statistically significantly higher than the control area (RR = 1.7; 95 percent CI = 1.1–2.7). The wide confidence interval includes values as low as 1.1 and as high as 2.7. The liver cancer rates in the other four reclaimed water areas do not differ from the control area (RR ranging from 0.9 in RW 3 to 1.4 in RW 2). Although RW 5 has the highest rate ratio, the pattern of rate ratios in the other four reclaimed water areas is inconsistent with a dose-response relationship between reclaimed water and liver cancer.[5]

For pancreas cancer and rectum cancer, the rate ratios indicate no association with reclaimed water. The rate ratios for these two cancer sites are close to 1.0, indicating the rates in the reclaimed water and control areas are nearly the same. All confidence intervals around the rate ratios for these two cancer sites include 1.0. The lack of a pattern in the rate ratios also indicates no association between the percentage of reclaimed water and pancreas and rectum cancer.

The rate of stomach cancer is statistically significantly higher in RW 2 than in the control area (RR = 1.29; 95 percent CI = 1.0–1.6). None of the other reclaimed water areas have rates significantly higher than the control area. It seems unlikely that the higher stomach cancer rate in RW 2 results from to a causal association between reclaimed water and stomach cancer for two reasons. First, RW 2 has the highest rate, but receives a very low percentage of reclaimed water (30-year average = 1.2 percent), making a causal association between reclaimed water and stomach cancer seem unlikely. Second, two areas (RW 4 and RW 5) that receive higher percentages of reclaimed water have stomach cancer rates lower than the control area.

---

[5]A dose-response threshold below which no effect will occur is toxicologically plausible. For most cancers, it is generally assumed that no such threshold exists. There are, however, known exceptions to this rule.

Mortality

The results of the mortality data analyses for a three-year period (1989–1991) are presented in Table 4.3. The mortality data were analyzed for two reasons: to evaluate the patterns of health outcomes other than cancers and to maintain methodologic consistency with the previous epidemiologic studies of the Montebello Forebay (Frerichs, 1981, 1982, 1983). For all deaths combined and each specific cause of death, we present the rate ratios and confidence intervals based on the parameters estimated by the Poisson regression models. These analyses statistically control for differences among the comparison groups in age, sex, and ethnicity. In reviewing these results, the reader should keep in mind that the analysis of the mortality data may present a biased view of the underlying rates of disease. Incidence of cancer and other diseases is considered to be a more reliable indicator of the effect of an environmental exposure for several reasons.[6] The number of deaths by cause can be found in Table F.2 for the five reclaimed water areas and the control area (Appendix F).

Table 4.3

Rate Ratios and Confidence Intervals for Mortality, Controlling for
Age, Sex, and Ethnicity, 1989–1991

Cause of Death	Area					
	RW 1	RW 2	RW 3	RW 4	RW 5	Control
All causes	1.05	1.19[a]	1.07	0.94	1.04	1.00
	(0.96–1.14)	(1.07-1.32)	(1.00-1.16)	(0.86-1.03)	(0.93-1.17)	
Cancer						
All sites	1.06	1.20[a]	1.12[a]	0.99	1.14[a]	1.00
	(0.97–1.15)	(1.04–1.37)	(1.02–1.23)	(0.89–1.11)	(1.03–1.26)	
Bladder	1.18	1.01	0.96	0.82	0.94	1.00
	(0.64–2.18)	(0.45–2.27)	(0.52–1.78)	(0.42–1.60)	(0.40–2.20)	
Colon	1.00	1.32	1.27	0.93	0.86	1.00
	(0.76–1.31)	(0.96–1.82)	(0.93–1.73)	(0.67–1.29)	(0.59–1.26)	
Esophagus	1.32	0.87	0.69	1.27	0.75	1.00
	(0.76–2.29)	(0.35–2.16)	(0.32–1.48)	(0.71–2.26)	(0.24–2.38)	
Kidney	0.87	1.37	0.56	0.66	0.51	1.00
	(0.50–1.51)	(0.76–2.46)	(0.27–1.14)	(0.35–1.23)	(0.20–1.28)	
Liver	1.10	1.19	0.90	0.86	1.40	1.00
	(0.69–1.73)	(0.74–1.92)	(0.58–1.39)	(0.48–1.54)	(0.88–2.24)	
Pancreas	1.01	1.21	1.14	0.89	1.25	1.00
	(0.71–1.43)	(0.77–1.92)	(0.79–1.66)	(0.58–1.38)	(0.84–1.85)	
Rectum	1.02	1.70	1.25	0.88	1.50	1.00
	(0.45–2.31)	(0.72–4.01)	(0.51–3.03)	(0.34–2.26)	(0.57–3.96)	
Stomach	1.24	1.71[a]	1.34	1.51	1.50	1.00
	(0.81–1.90)	(1.16–2.53)	(0.89–2.03)	(0.96–2.37)	(0.99–2.26)	
Heart Disease	1.01	1.19[a]	1.09	0.93	1.02	1.00
	(0.91–1.12)	(1.07–1.33)	(0.99–1.20)	(0.83–1.05)	(0.89–1.18)	
Cerebrovascular Disease	1.16	1.09	1.14	0.92	1.00	1.00
	(1.00–1.35)	(0.89–1.33)	(0.97–1.34)	(0.74–1.14)	(0.81–1.23)	
All Other	1.05	1.20[a]	1.02	0.93	1.02	1.00
	(0.95–1.16)	(1.06–1.36)	(0.93–1.11)	(0.83–1.04)	(0.88–1.18)	

[a]Statistically significantly different from 1.0 (p < 0.05).

---

[6]These reasons are listed in "Selection of Health Outcomes" in Chapter Three.

Although death rates for all causes were not hypothesized to be related to reclaimed water, they were analyzed as part of the assessment. RW 2 has a statistically significantly higher death rate from all causes than the control area (RR = 1.2, 95 percent CI = 1.1–1.3). The death rates in the other four reclaimed water areas are similar to the control area.

Mortality rates for all cancer sites combined are significantly higher in three RW areas (RW 2, RW 3, and RW 5) than in the control area (Table 4.3). This category was also not hypothesized to be related to reclaimed water. The rate ratios are 1.20, 1.12, and 1.14, respectively, and their 95 percent confidence intervals do not include 1.0, indicating that they are statistically significantly higher than 1.0. The death rates from all cancers in RW 1 and RW 4 are similar to the control area.

Stomach cancer death rates are higher in all the reclaimed water areas than in the control area (Table 4.3). Rate ratios range from a low of 1.24 in RW 1 to a high of 1.71 in RW 2. The rate in RW 2 is statistically significantly higher than the rate in the control area (95 percent CI = 1.16–2.53). Although all five of the rate ratios are greater than 1.0, the pattern is not consistent with a dose-response relationship between reclaimed water and stomach cancer deaths (i.e., the rate ratios do not increase with increasing percentages of reclaimed water).

Death rates from cancer of the bladder, colon, esophagus, kidney, liver, pancreas, and rectum do not differ significantly between the reclaimed water areas and the control area (Table 4.3). Of the rate ratios for these seven sites, some are higher than 1.0 and some are lower than 1.0. All of the confidence intervals include 1.0, indicating no statistically significant differences between the reclaimed water areas and the control area. The smallest rate ratio is for kidney cancer deaths in RW 5 (RR = 0.51; 95 percent CI = 0.20–1.28). The largest rate ratio is for rectum cancer deaths in RW 2 (RR = 1.70; 95 percent CI = 0.72–4.01). Most of the remaining rate ratios have values between 0.75 and 1.5.[7] The rate ratios do not exhibit the patterns that would be expected if there was a dose-response relationship between reclaimed water and these causes of death.

The rectum cancer death rate was of some interest because of previous findings. Earlier epidemiologic studies reported an increased mortality rate from rectum cancer in areas receiving reclaimed water (Frerichs et al., 1981, 1983). In the current study, the rectal cancer death rate is higher in the area with the highest percentage of reclaimed water (RW 5) than in the control area (RR = 1.50), but this difference is not statistically significant (95 percent CI = 0.57–3.96). In the current study, as in the earlier studies, the rate ratio based on *incidence* data, however, does not indicate a higher rate of newly diagnosed cases of rectum cancer in RW 5 (RR = 0.97). Because

---

[7]Information derived from death certificates on liver cancer may be less reliable than for other cancer sites. Because the liver is a frequent metastatic site for other primary cancers, and the distinction between primary and secondary liver cancer is often not made on the death certificate, liver cancer may be overestimated from cause of death information.

incidence data are considered to be a more reliable indicator of geographic patterns of occurrence, the mortality finding is of interest, but not meaningful.

The rate ratios for mortality from heart disease range from 0.93 (RW 4) to 1.19 (RW 2), for mortality from cerebrovascular disease from 0.92 (RW 4) to 1.16 (RW 1), and for mortality from all other causes from 0.93 (RW 4) to 1.20 (RW 2). Although some of these rate ratios are statistically significantly different from 1.0, they occurred in areas with low percentages of reclaimed water. In addition, these causes of death were not hypothesized to be related to reclaimed water.

Infectious Disease Incidence

Infectious agents that have been implicated as the cause of waterborne outbreaks of illness in the United States or other countries were analyzed as part of our epidemiologic assessment. We conducted separate analyses for four diseases: giardia, hepatitis A, salmonella, and shigella. Several other infectious diseases infrequently reported to health departments were analyzed as a single category: typhoid fever, amebiasis, meningitis of unspecified origin, leptospirosis, cholera, and gastroenteritis.[8] The results of these analyses are shown in Table 4.4. The number of cases by infectious disease category can be found in Table F.3 for each of the reclaimed water areas and the control area (Appendix F).

Table 4.4

Rate Ratios and Confidence Intervals for Infectious Disease Incidence,
Controlling for Age, Sex, and Ethnicity, 1989–1990

Disease	Area					
	RW 1	RW 2	RW 3	RW 4	RW 5	Control
Giardia	1.05 (0.72–1.52)	1.43[a] (1.03–1.99)	0.80 (0.56–1.16)	0.76 (0.51–1.12)	0.68 (0.38–1.20)	1.00
Hepatitis A	1.16 (0.87–1.54)	1.44[a] (1.04–1.99)	1.40[a] (1.05–1.85)	1.10 (0.73–1.67)	1.12 (0.83–1.51)	1.00
Salmonella	0.91 (0.71–1.18)	1.19 (0.94–1.51)	0.93 (0.72–1.19)	1.17 (0.86–1.60)	0.83 (0.54–1.28)	1.00
Shigella	1.42[a] (1.14–1.77)	1.31[a] (1.03–1.68)	1.28[a] (1.04–1.58)	1.02 (0.74–1.39)	1.12 (0.82–1.53)	1.00
Other[b]	1.22 (0.79–1.89)	1.10 (0.72–1.68)	0.91 (0.55–1.52)	0.76 (0.40–1.43)	1.36 (0.79–2.35)	1.00
All of the above[c]	1.16 (0.97–1.39)	1.32[a] (1.15–1.52)	1.09 (0.95–1.26)	0.99 (0.83–1.17)	0.98 (0.79–1.23)	1.00

[a]Statistically significantly different from 1.0 ($p < 0.05$).

[b]Includes typhoid fever, amebiasis, unspecified meningitis, leptospirosis, cholera, and gastroenteritis.

[c]Includes all infectious diseases shown in the first five lines of the table.

---

[8]Only one case of cholera and no cases of leptospirosis were reported to the Los Angeles County Department of Health Services in 1989 and 1990.

There is considerable variation in the magnitude of the rate ratios for giardia among the five reclaimed water areas, with the values ranging from 0.7 to 1.4 (Table 4.4). RW 2 has a statistically significantly higher rate than the control area (RR = 1.4, 95 percent CI = 1.03–1.99). Of the other four areas, three (RW 3, RW 4, and RW 5) have rate ratios less than 1.0, and RW 1 has a rate ratio greater than 1.0. The confidence intervals around these four rate ratios include 1.0, indicating no differences. There is also no indication of increasing rates with increasing percentages of reclaimed water.

The rate of hepatitis A is statistically significantly higher in RW 2 and RW 3 than in the control area (Table 4.4). Although all five rate ratios for hepatitis A are greater than 1.0, the pattern of results does not indicate a dose-response relationship between reclaimed water and hepatitis A. The rate ratios for hepatitis A are higher in the areas with less reclaimed water (RW 2 and RW 3) than those with more (RW 4 and RW 5).

The rate ratios for salmonella infection do not indicate differences in the rates between the reclaimed water and control areas (Table 4.4). All five confidence intervals include 1.0 and rate ratios range in value from 0.8 (RW 5) to 1.2 (RW 2) with no indication of a dose-response relationship.

The rate ratios for shigella indicate higher rates for those living in areas with lower percentages of reclaimed water (Table 4.4). The three areas with the least reclaimed water in their supplies (RW 1, 2, and 3) have rate ratios statistically significantly greater than 1.0 (RR = 1.4, 1.3, and 1.3, respectively), whereas the two areas with more reclaimed water (RW 4 and 5) have rate ratios close to 1.0. This pattern of results does not support the hypothesis of an association between reclaimed water and shigella infection.

The pattern of rate ratios for the "other" infectious diseases do not indicate a relationship between reclaimed water and these uncommon diseases (Table 4.4). Because the areas with less reclaimed water (RW 1 and RW 2) have higher rate ratios than those with more (RW 3 and RW 4), their occurrence appears to be unrelated to the percentage of reclaimed water in the water supply.

The rate ratios for the "all of the above" category in Table 4.4 clearly show that, as a group, these infectious diseases are not reported more frequently among those living in areas with higher percentages of reclaimed water in their water supplies. The pattern goes in the opposite direction; those in areas with more reclaimed water have rate ratios close to 1.0, whereas those in areas with less reclaimed water have rate ratios greater than 1.0 (RW 1, RW 2, and RW 3).

SENSITIVITY ANALYSES

The cancer, mortality, and infectious disease data were analyzed using two alternative models to assess the sensitivity of the results to the variables included. The first model controls for age and sex only and the second model controls for age, sex, race/ethnicity, and income. The rate ratios and 95 percent confidence intervals for these two models are shown for cancer incidence in Appendix G, mortality in Appendix H, and infectious diseases in Appendix I.

The overall pattern of results and the magnitude of the estimates remain generally unchanged by the alternative models, indicating that the patterns observed in Tables 4.2–4.4 are not explained by the distribution of the Hispanic population or income. Most of the statistically significant results remain statistically significant under the two alternative models. The elevated incidence rate for liver cancer in the RW 5 area is significant under all three models. For a more detailed discussion of these results, see Appendices G, H, and I.

To assess the sensitivity of the results to the choice of control locations, we compared the three separate control locations with the reclaimed water areas and with one another. In general, these comparisons did not reveal any differences among the control locations that would affect the conclusions of the study. The results of these analyses are summarized in Appendix J.

Chapter Five

DISCUSSION

The epidemiologic study reported here investigated the rate of health outcomes in the Montebello Forebay of Los Angeles County from 1987 to 1991, almost 30 years after groundwater recharge with some reclaimed water was initiated. Previous epidemiologic studies concluded that the level of reclaimed water used for recharge in the Montebello Forebay from 1962 to 1980 had no detectable impact on human health (Nellor et al., 1984; Frerichs et al., 1981, 1982, 1983). This report documents another evaluation of the patterns of selected health outcomes under circumstances that differ from the earlier epidemiologic studies in three ways. First, the time period evaluated by the current study (1987–1991) is almost 30 years after groundwater recharge with some reclaimed water began. This means that this study can evaluate longer-term exposure than the earlier epidemiologic studies, which were conducted less than 20 years after groundwater recharge with reclaimed water was initiated (Frerichs et al., 1981, 1982, 1983). Second, the percentage of reclaimed water is higher in many Montebello Forebay water supplies because the volume of reclaimed water used to recharge the groundwater basin increased substantially between 1980 and 1990. Third, the population receiving some reclaimed water is almost twice the size of that studied earlier. This increase is explained primarily by additional geographic areas using groundwater containing reclaimed water. These three factors increase the likelihood of finding an effect of reclaimed water on the health of those consuming it, if such an effect exists.

SUMMARY OF RESULTS

This study tested the hypothesis of an association between reclaimed water and a broad range of biologically plausible health outcomes for the five-year period from 1987 to 1991. The health outcomes included cancer incidence (all cancers and cancer of the bladder, colon, esophagus, kidney, liver, pancreas, rectum, and stomach), mortality (deaths due to all causes, heart disease, stroke, all cancer, and the eight specific cancer sites), and infectious diseases (giardia, hepatitis A, salmonella, shigella, and several less common diseases). Compared to the control area, some areas receiving reclaimed water had higher rates and others had lower rates for the health outcomes. The pattern of results does not support the hypothesis of a causal relationship between reclaimed water and cancer, mortality, or infectious disease. If reclaimed water led to an increase in disease, the pattern of results would be expected to show evidence of a dose-response relationship in which the rates of disease are higher in areas with more reclaimed water. This is not what we found.

Statistically Significant Results

Statistical significance is often used in epidemiology and other disciplines to highlight the "most important" results. Although statistical significance should not be the only criterion used in judging which results are most important, its widespread acceptance as a standard of importance justifies some discussion of its occurrence and meaning in the context of this study.

Liver Cancer Incidence. The liver cancer rate in RW 5 was statistically significantly higher than in the control area. This result is of special interest because it occurred in the area with the highest percentage of reclaimed water. Three possible explanations for the higher rate of liver cancer in RW 5 should be considered: reclaimed water, differences other than reclaimed water, and random occurrence.

The *first possible explanation* for the higher rate of liver cancer in RW 5 is that the association between reclaimed water and liver cancer is causal. The evaluation of this possibility cites the available evidence.

Strength: The rate ratio for liver cancer in RW 5 is 1.73, reflecting a moderately increased rate compared to the control area. Although this is the largest rate ratio observed in this study, in general, rate ratios less than 2.0 are interpreted cautiously. If it were based on a large number of cases, the size of the rate ratio might be more compelling. It is based, however, on 34 cases of liver cancer occurring over a five-year period—an average of seven cases per year diagnosed in a population of 116,000 people.

Consistency: Little evidence from other studies supports a causal relationship between reclaimed water and liver cancer. One ecologic study of the health effects of chlorinated surface water reported elevated rates of liver cancer mortality (Marienfeld et al., 1986).[1]

Temporality: Use of reclaimed water for groundwater recharge began in 1962, so the presence of reclaimed water in the Montebello Forebay water supplies preceded the occurrence of liver cancer cases in 1987–1991. Because information on exposure to home tap water for each of the liver cancer cases is not available, it is impossible to verify how much reclaimed water each person who developed liver cancer actually drank prior to onset of the disease.

Biologic gradient: The pattern of rate ratios in the five reclaimed water areas does not suggest a dose-response relationship between reclaimed water and liver cancer. RW 5 had the highest rate ratio and RW 2 had the second highest.

---

[1]As noted in Chapter Four, however, information on liver cancer derived from death certificates may be less reliable than that from other sites because of poor data quality. Other studies of chlorinated surface water included in the literature review either did not analyze data on liver cancer or did not observe an association between liver cancer and chlorinated surface water.

Plausibility and coherence: The liver has been found to be susceptible to ingested carcinogenic compounds, such as alcohol and aflatoxin (Higginson et al., 1992). No presumptive carcinogenic action, however, was detected in the samples of reclaimed water tested during the Health Effects Study; mutagenicity was found to be intermediate between the high mutagenicity of surface runoff and the low mutagenicity of imported Colorado River water (Nellor et al., 1984, Robeck et al., 1987). Therefore, it seems implausible that drinking reclaimed water influences the rate of liver cancer.

The *second possible explanation* for the higher rate of liver cancer is that differences other than reclaimed water exist between RW 5 and the control area that affect the rate of liver cancer. Known risk factors for liver cancer include viral infections (hepatitis B and hepatitis C), chronic alcohol abuse, and alcoholic cirrhosis (Higginson et al., 1992). We could not control for these factors in our analysis and therefore they might account for the higher rate of liver cancer in RW 5.

The *third possible explanation* for the elevated liver cancer rate ratio is random occurrence. Forty rate ratios were calculated in the analysis for site-specific cancer incidence; of these only two were statistically significant. This is exactly the number of statistically significant results that would be expected to occur by chance alone.[2] Therefore, the liver cancer result may be explained entirely by chance.

Stomach Cancer Incidence. The significant stomach cancer rate ratio (based on 91 cases over a five-year period or an average of 18 cases per year) occurred in the area with the second lowest percentage of reclaimed water (RW 2). The areas with the most reclaimed water have the lowest rate ratios for stomach cancer, 0.99 (RW 4) and 0.85 (RW 5). The hypothesis of a dose-response relationship between reclaimed water and stomach cancer is not supported by the fact that the area with little exposure to reclaimed water has a higher rate ratio than the areas with much higher exposure. Known risk factors for stomach cancer include dietary factors and the presence of the bacterium Helicobacter pylori in the stomach (Higginson et al., 1992). These or other factors may explain the elevated rate in RW 2.

Mortality. Significantly elevated death rates from stomach cancer were observed in RW 2. These results are based on 39 stomach cancer deaths over a three-year period. Given that RW 2 receives a very low percentage of reclaimed water, it is unlikely that the higher stomach cancer death rate can be attributed to reclaimed water.

Infectious Disease. All six significantly elevated rates of infectious disease occurred in the three areas with the lowest percentages of reclaimed water—RW 1, RW 2, and RW 3. Higher rates of shigella were found in all three of these areas (based on 128, 107, and 127 cases over a two-year period, respectively) compared to the control area. Higher rates of hepatitis A in RW 2 and RW 3 and an elevated rate of giardia in RW 2 were also observed. If reclaimed water were responsible for the higher rates, the areas with more reclaimed water would also be expected to have higher rates. This was not the case.

---

[2]The number of results expected to be statistically significant by chance alone can be calculated as the alpha level (0.05) times the number of statistical tests (40), or (0.05 × 40 = 2).

All Outcomes. When a large number of statistical tests are conducted, a certain proportion would be expected to achieve statistical significance by chance alone. In comparing the observed and expected number of significant associations, we found that data on cancer incidence and mortality yielded the expected number of significant results. However, we observed more than the expected number of significant results in the infectious disease data. Forty statistical tests to compare cancer incidence rates were conducted.[3] Of these, two were statistically significantly higher than 1.0, exactly the number that would be expected by chance alone: 5 percent (the alpha level) of 40. Two of the 50 rate ratios for ten causes of death are statistically significantly higher than 1.0.[4] This is the number of statistically significant results that would be expected by chance alone: 5 percent (the alpha level) of 50. For infectious diseases, 25 statistical tests were conducted, of which six indicated rate ratios were statistically significantly higher than 1.0.[5] Thus, for infectious diseases, there appears to be an excess of significant results: only one or two would be expected based on 5 percent (the alpha level) of 25. These figures may indicate that the higher rates observed for cancer and mortality are chance occurrences that may not be caused by any exposure or characteristic in the populations.

Trends in Results

It is noteworthy that the rates in the reclaimed water areas are higher than in the control area more than half the time (i.e., more than half of the rate ratios are greater than 1.0). If the rates in the reclaimed water and control areas were equal, we would expect to find about the same number of rate ratios above and below 1.0 (i.e., about 50 percent above and 50 percent below). Instead, we find the following: 29 of the 40 cancer rate ratios are higher than 1.0 and 11 are lower; 32 of the 50 mortality rate ratios are higher than 1.0 and 18 are lower; 17 of the 25 infectious disease rate ratios are higher than 1.0 and 8 are lower. Thus, for cancer, almost three-fourths of the rate ratios are above 1.0, whereas for mortality and infectious diseases, about two-thirds are above 1.0.

The slightly higher rates tend to occur in areas with lower percentages of reclaimed water. If higher rates of disease were being caused by reclaimed water, the elevated rate ratios would be expected to occur more frequently in those areas with *more* reclaimed water. The higher rate ratios, however, do not occur more frequently in those areas with more reclaimed water. The area with the second lowest percentage of reclaimed water (RW 2) has many more rate ratios above 1.0 than would be ex-

---

[3]The five tests for "all cancer" were excluded from this discussion because we did not hypothesize a priori that the rate of all cancers might be affected by reclaimed water. Rather, we analyzed data on all cancers to characterize the general health status of these populations.

[4]The 15 tests for all causes of death, all cancer deaths, and all other causes of death were excluded from this discussion because our a priori hypotheses related to the effects of reclaimed water did not include these broad categories of death.

[5]The five tests for all selected infectious diseases were excluded from this discussion because they are based on the other five categories collapsed together and thus would be redundant.

pected: seven of eight cancer outcomes, nine of ten mortality outcomes, and all of five infectious disease outcomes. On the other hand, the area with the second highest percentage of reclaimed water (RW 4) has fewer rate ratios above 1.0 than would be expected: four of eight cancer outcomes, two of ten mortality outcomes, and three of five infectious disease outcomes. The other three areas (RW 1, RW 3, and RW 5) have slightly more rate ratios above 1.0 than would be expected. These findings are probably attributable to differences between the reclaimed water and control areas that are completely unrelated to reclaimed water. Given the ecologic nature of this study, we are unable to investigate what these differences might be.

Evidence Related to Causality

Chapter Four defined the characteristics of an association that might support the hypothesis of causality—strength, consistency, temporality, biologic gradient, plausibility, and coherence (Rothman, 1986; Hill, 1965). Each of these topics will be discussed briefly relative to the overall study results.

Strength. Most rate ratios in this study were between 0.75 and 1.50; the largest was 1.74. Rate ratios in this range are considered moderate to small in magnitude and would not be considered suggestive of causality unless several other criteria pointed in that direction.

Consistency. The study indicates that reclaimed water does not have any detectable effect on human health. This conclusion is consistent with the results of water quality studies and previous epidemiologic studies of the health effects of reclaimed water.

Temporality. The criterion of temporality has been met in this study—the data on exposure to reclaimed water used in the analysis were based on a time period preceding the health effects data. The availability of historical information on percentage of reclaimed water in the water supplies in the Montebello Forebay allows the exposure and outcome data to be "lagged" appropriately by the hypothesized induction period.

Biologic gradient. This aspect, referred to as the "dose-response relationship," has been discussed extensively in our study results. The patterns of results are not what would be expected if reclaimed water were causing a health effect; rates of disease are not higher in areas with higher percentages of reclaimed water.

Plausibility. The absence of biologic and chemical agents in reclaimed water is biologically consistent with the finding of no consistently increased rates of disease in areas with reclaimed water.

Coherence. The results of the study do not conflict with what is known about reclaimed water and the diseases included in the analysis.

COMPARISON OF RESULTS WITH OTHER STUDIES

Previous Epidemiologic Studies of the Montebello Forebay

Elevated rates of mortality resulting from rectum cancer were observed consistently in the epidemiologic studies of the Montebello Forebay populations completed in the early 1980s (Frerichs et al., 1981, 1982, 1983). Further work, however, revealed that the incidence of rectum cancer (i.e., newly diagnosed cases of rectum cancer) was not higher in the reclaimed water area (Frerichs et al., 1983). In the current study, we observed patterns of rectum cancer incidence and mortality similar to those in these earlier studies. In the area with the highest percentage of reclaimed water (RW 5), the rate ratio for mortality due to rectum cancer was 1.50, indicating a higher rate than in the control area, but not significantly so. The rate ratio for incidence of rectum cancer, however, was 0.97, a rate about the same as in the control area. Although the findings in the earlier studies and the current study are hard to compare because of differences in analytic methods, the pattern is consistent. Because we consider the patterns of cancer incidence to be a better measure of rate than mortality, these results indicate there is not an higher rate of rectum cancer in the area with the highest percentage of reclaimed water.[6]

Epidemiologic Studies of Chlorinated Surface Water and Cancer

We compare the results of the current study to epidemiologic studies of chlorinated surface water. Although these are not studies of reclaimed water that has been intentionally reused, most are studies of reclaimed water that has been reused unintentionally, as in communities being served surface water downstream from industrial and municipal centers. Several epidemiologic studies suggest an association between chlorinated surface water and increased incidence of bladder and rectum cancer. Associations between cancers at other sites and chlorinated surface water have also been reported, but with inconsistent results. In the current study, elevated rates of bladder or rectum cancers (based on incidence data) were not found for the reclaimed water areas. The rate ratios ranged from 0.85 to 1.03 for bladder cancer, and from 0.89 to 1.09 for rectum cancer, indicating that the rates of developing these two cancers are not higher in the reclaimed water areas than in the control area. The rate ratios for the area with the highest percentage of reclaimed water (RW 5) were 1.03 for bladder cancer and 0.97 for rectum cancer.[7] It thus appears that the results

---

[6]As in the earlier report, we consider changes in incidence more sensitive to environmental exposures, for three reasons. First, incidence would be expected to change in response to an environmental exposure earlier than would mortality. Second, incidence is not affected by survival factors. Third, the incidence data are based on diagnostic information from patient medical records, in addition to cause-of-death information from death certificates.

The higher mortality caused by rectum cancer without a corresponding increase in incidence may be explained by different coding practices by physicians in that area (Frerichs et al., 1983). In one study area, physicians may have attributed deaths to the category coded as rectum cancer more liberally than in the other study areas.

[7]RW 5 is the only area in the Montebello Forebay that received an average of more than 5 percent reclaimed water in its water supply in the mid to late 1960s. The average percentage of reclaimed water in the water supplies of RW 5 has increased steadily since 1962 when reclaimed water was first used for groundwater recharge.

from previous epidemiologic studies of cancer and chlorinated surface water were not replicated in the current research.

ECOLOGIC STUDY DESIGN

The study described in this report was conducted using an ecologic study design, and understanding the design's features is important because it affects the way in which the study results can be interpreted. [This discussion draws heavily from the overview by Walter (1991a).] The unique feature of an ecologic study is that the unit of analysis is a group of individuals, whereas other epidemiologic study designs analyze data on individuals. Higher disease rates in populations with higher exposure are interpreted as an indication of a possible causal association. Ecologic studies are important tools in etiologic research and public health surveillance. They evaluate potential public health problems rapidly and determine whether a hypothesis is worth pursuing.

Limitations of Ecologic Study Design

Among the many issues that might affect the quality of an ecologic study (Walter, 1991b) are quality of the numerator data, quality of the denominator data, accuracy of exposure data, induction period for disease development, population mobility, and ecologic fallacy. The possible effect of each of these on this study is discussed below.

Quality of numerator (health outcomes) data. Each health outcome must be defined and recorded in a consistent manner, and health outcomes for the area or group under study must be ascertained completely. In this study, the data on cancer incidence are of high quality; the mortality and infectious disease data must be interpreted somewhat more cautiously. Cancer incidence rates were estimated from data from a high-quality cancer registry, the University of Southern California Cancer Surveillance Program (CSP). The CSP documents all cancers diagnosed in Los Angeles County using active surveillance methods. Mortality rates were derived from death certificate data. Although registration of deaths is virtually 100 percent complete in the United States, cause of death or place of residence at the time of death may be not be accurate. Infectious disease rates were based on the cases reported to the Los Angeles County Department of Health Services. Reporting rates may differ for different diseases. Despite the possible problems associated with mortality data and infectious disease data, however, there is no reason to suspect that quality of the mortality data or reporting rates for infectious diseases differ between the reclaimed water areas and the control area. Therefore, although the cancer data probably reflect actual occurrence more accurately and completely than do the data on mortality and infectious disease, all three data sources are likely unbiased with respect to the study areas.

Quality of denominator (population) data. An ecologic study requires an accurate count of the number of people at risk of developing a disease. For this study, population counts by age, sex, and ethnicity were derived from the 1990 U.S. Census. In the calculation of rates, these counts represent the population at risk of disease, that is, the denominator. In the United States, the counts from the decennial censuses conducted by the U.S. Bureau of the Census represent the most accurate estimates of the resident population available. In these surveys, every household in the United States receives a mailed questionnaire asking the householder to enumerate the people living there. Response rates are high because nonrespondents are contacted by census personnel.

Accuracy of exposure data. Exposure to reclaimed water was estimated in this study using a state-of-the-art model based on hydrogeologic and statistical theory. Input to the model consisted of actual data on the operating parameters of the water systems serving residential customers. The results of the model were validated to the extent possible. Nonetheless, the methods yield approximate measures, subject to some measurement error. Consequently, percentages of reclaimed water were used to classify census tracts into five broad exposure categories for the analyses.

In an ecologic study, it is assumed that a single exposure value can be assigned to all people in a subgroup (Walter, 1991b), which in this study was the census tract. The assumption of homogeneous exposure for all residents of a census tract may not in fact hold. Individual exposure to tap water may vary greatly for several reasons. Some people may drink some or all of their tap water away from home (i.e., at work or at other locations). Others may not drink tap water at any location, drinking bottled water or other beverages all of the time. In the 1980 survey of women living in the reclaimed water area of the Montebello Forebay, 28 percent reported buying bottled water and 23 percent reported not drinking tap water (Frerichs, 1982). It is possible that during the period of the current study (1987–1991), an even higher proportion of people bought bottled water or did not drink tap water, given the widespread attention water quality has received during the last decade. In addition to water source, the volume of water consumed (i.e., number of glasses per day) is a factor influencing exposure. All of these factors make it unlikely that a single exposure measure for a census tract accurately reflects the variation in consumption that is likely. If it can be assumed that factors influencing consumption patterns are fairly similar in all census tracts, however, the census tract–level measure of exposure may accurately reflect how the average exposure level of one census tract compares with other census tracts.

Induction period for disease development. The induction period has been defined as "the period of time from causal action until disease initiation" (Rothman, 1986). Based on this definition, any disease with multiple causes (which includes virtually all diseases) cannot be said to have a long or short induction period, because the length of the induction period depends on the causal factor being considered. In carcinogenesis, causes that act in the early stages of the disease process have been called initiators and those that act in the later stages are called promotors. Although cancer has been characterized as a disease with a long induction period, if an initiator-promotor model holds, the induction period for the promotor causes may be shorter than for the initiator causes (Rothman, 1986). Assumptions related to an induction period are not easy to prove or disprove because the role of chemical exposures and their timing in the induction of cancer are not well understood (Moolgavkar, 1994).

The timing of exposure relative to the occurrence of disease must be considered in interpreting the results. The induction periods for cancers may be long (decades) or short (years) and are poorly understood. Their length undoubtedly varies by cause and by cancer site. The induction periods for infectious diseases are known to be quite short (days, weeks, or months). Because no suspected or confirmed carcinogen has been identified in reclaimed water, no specific assumptions can be made regarding the disease model and the length of the induction period. If the induction period is assumed to be long (i.e., 20–30 years), the percentage of reclaimed water in the 1960s and 1970s would influence the rates most. If the induction period is assumed to be short (i.e., 5–10 years), however, the percentage of reclaimed water in the 1980s would be most influential. In this study, because the percentages of reclaimed water in the 1960s and in the 1980s are highly correlated, using the exposure measure based on 1960–1980 or 1960–1990 makes little difference in the analysis or interpretation of the results.

Effect of population mobility. Half or more of the people living in the Los Angeles County area move over a five-year period. Based on 1990 census data, 51 percent of people living in the reclaimed water areas reported that they had lived in the same residence five years earlier (in 1985). In the control area, fewer (45 percent) had resided in the same place for five years or longer. These percentages are representative of Los Angeles County as a whole (47 percent). The high mobility rate implies that many people in the reclaimed water have been exposed to many different water supplies during their lifetime, of which perhaps only the most recent contained reclaimed water.

Exactly how the mobility of the Montebello Forebay population might affect the results of this study cannot be estimated. If the induction period for a disease is long, the high population mobility rates in the Montebello Forebay may make interpretation of the study results difficult. If the induction period for a disease is short, however, these high rates of population mobility (in- and out-migration) will not affect interpretation of the results. In general, people who move away from the Montebello Forebay area after living there for many years will not be included in the analysis, whereas people who recently moved into the Montebello Forebay will be included. If long-time residents move out of the area, the proportion of people who have been "exposed" to reclaimed water for a long period of time will decrease. As new residents move into the area to replace those who have moved out, the proportion of people who have been "exposed" to reclaimed water for a short period of time will increase. Although out-migration will not bias estimates of exposure effects (assuming out-migration is independent of disease status), it reduces statistical power by reducing the sample size of exposed persons (Hatch et al., 1990). Including people who recently moved into the area, however, will result in exposure misclassification and may weaken estimates of effect (Polissar, 1980). As pointed out above, however, little is known about the induction period and timing associated with the carcinogenic process, making a judgment regarding the effect of mobility on the results difficult.

Ecologic fallacy. A major limitation of ecologic studies is the possibility of bias in the estimation of the effect under study. The problem known as "ecologic fallacy" arises when a conclusion regarding associations at the individual level are based on an analysis of group-level data. In ecologic studies, no information is available on the distribution of exposure and outcomes at the individual level, so that there is no information on whether the individual who develops a health outcome has ever had a particular exposure. The bias that may result from analyzing group-level data can result in the ecologic association seeming to be stronger or weaker than the true association at the individual level. In most studies, however, the bias increases the magnitude of the true association (Morgenstern, 1982).

The results of this ecologic study may be subject to the bias associated with ecologic fallacy. Because information on exposure to reclaimed water and occurrence of diseases is not available on individuals, the association between the two is assessed using census-tract-level data, rather than individual-level data. The information on exposure is based on the percentage of reclaimed water in the water supply of each census tract, rather than how much reclaimed water each individual consumes. The rates of various health outcomes are also estimated at the group level, in this case for the population living in the census tract. The results of this study, therefore, accurately represent the relationship between reclaimed water and health outcomes at the group level, but may be less accurate in representing the association at the individual level.

Confounding factors. In this ecologic study, some important risk factors that might confound the results could not be controlled for. We controlled for differences between the reclaimed water and control areas in three of the most important determinants of disease risk (i.e., risk factors): age, sex, and ethnicity. Information on other important risk factors, however, was not available at the individual or census-tract level. Table 5.1 lists factors that have been associated with occurrence of the cancers in this study. These characteristics were assumed to be distributed equally on average across the reclaimed water and control areas. If the distribution of these factors differs, the observed patterns may be the result of these or other uncontrolled factors.

Advantages of Ecologic Study Design

If the results of the study are interpreted cautiously, an ecologic study has several advantages over other types of epidemiologic studies—the ability to study large populations, to investigate a large number of health outcomes in a single study, and to address questions related to environmental exposure that would be difficult to study with other designs (Walter, 1991a).

Ecologic studies allow complete evaluation of the health status of large populations. This study includes information on health outcomes over a five-year period in a population of 1.6 million people, representing 18 percent of Los Angeles County. A total of 25,104 cancers, 26,385 deaths, and 2679 cases of infectious disease were analyzed. Other epidemiologic study designs usually focus on a small subgroup of people.

Table 5.1

Risk Factors Associated with Selected Cancer Sites

Site of Cancer	Risk Factors
Bladder	Occupational exposure to dyes, tobacco, parasitic infection (schistosomiasis), artificial sweeteners
Colon	Family history, diet (high fat, low fiber, little fresh produce), ulcerative colitis, alcohol (weak association)
Esophagus	Family history, alcohol, tobacco, diet (little fresh produce)
Kidney	Tobacco, family history, overweight
Liver	Viral infections (hepatitis B and C), aflatoxin, alcohol, cirrhosis, oral contraceptives
Pancreas	Tobacco, diabetes, diet (high fat, little fresh produce)
Rectum	Family history, diet (high fat, low fiber, little fresh produce), ulcerative colitis, alcohol (weak association)
Stomach	Blood type, family history, certain foods (smoked, salted, fried, pickled), alcohol (weak association), tobacco (weak association), infection/presence of *Helicobacter pylori*

SOURCE: Higginson et al. (1992).

Because ecologic studies rely on existing data, a large number of health outcomes can be evaluated in a single study. The current study analyzed data on 9 cancer sites, 13 causes of death, and 6 infectious diseases. With other epidemiologic study designs, only one health outcome is usually studied. Focusing on one outcome is appropriate if evidence from previous studies supports the hypothesis of an association between the exposure and a specific outcome. Previous studies, however, have not suggested an association between reclaimed water and any particular health outcome. A broad-based investigation of many outcomes, therefore, seemed to be the best approach.

Ecologic study designs are often used in epidemiology to take a first look at the possible health effects of an environmental exposure. They are less expensive and time-consuming than other types of studies, because they rely on available morbidity, mortality, and census data. As pointed out above, ecologic studies often include data on large populations, allowing hypotheses regarding extremely uncommon events to be tested. In addition, hypotheses regarding numerous health outcomes can be investigated in a single study. For these reasons, an ecologic design is often preferred over other study designs to investigate health questions related to environmental exposures.

CONCLUSIONS

This epidemiologic study concludes that almost 30 years after groundwater recharge with some reclaimed water began, the rates of cancer, mortality, and infectious disease are similar in the area of Los Angeles County receiving some reclaimed water and a control area not receiving any reclaimed water. Rates of these health outcomes are also similar in areas receiving higher and lower percentages of reclaimed water. The analysis included routinely collected data on cancer incidence (all cancers, and cancer of the bladder, colon, esophagus, kidney, liver, pancreas, rectum, and stomach), mortality (deaths due to all causes, heart disease, stroke, all cancer and the eight specific cancer sites), and infectious diseases (giardia, hepatitis A, salmonella, shigella, and several less common diseases). There were few instances in which rates of disease or death were significantly higher in areas receiving reclaimed water than in the control area. Regions with less reclaimed water tended to have higher rates of adverse health outcomes than regions with more reclaimed water, leading to the conclusion that the observed higher rates were probably due either to chance or to unmeasured factors unrelated to reclaimed water exposure. A significantly higher incidence rate of liver cancer was observed in the area with the highest percentage of reclaimed water. Because there is no biologic or epidemiologic evidence to suggest a relationship between reclaimed water and liver cancer, this result is most likely explained by factors unrelated to reclaimed water or by chance occurrence.

The limitations of epidemiologic methods make drawing definitive conclusions about the effects of reclaimed water on health difficult. Personal characteristics that might affect disease rates—such as smoking, alcohol consumption, and occupational exposure—were assumed to be equal in the reclaimed water and control areas, but could not be controlled in the analysis. If the distribution of these factors differs substantially between the reclaimed water and control areas, the pattern of results may be attributable to these differences or to other uncontrolled factors. In addition, actual exposure to reclaimed water may differ from that estimated because of time spent away from home and consumption of bottled water and other beverages. Finally, the high population mobility in Los Angeles County may make detecting an effect more difficult. Despite its limitations, the results of this epidemiologic study provide no evidence that reclaimed water has an adverse effect on health.

FUTURE RESEARCH

This epidemiologic assessment provides abundant and useful information on how the rates of cancer, death, and disease in five areas receiving increasing levels of reclaimed water compare with those in a control area not receiving any reclaimed water. Several important questions related to the health effects of reclaimed water, however, remain unanswered. First, how do factors that might affect the rate of cancer, death, and disease (e.g., smoking, alcohol consumption, occupational exposures) compare in the reclaimed water and control areas? Second, does exposure to reclaimed water (i.e., consumption of home tap water) differ between the reclaimed water and control areas? Studying these two questions would address some of the limitations of the ecologic study described in this report. Third, are rates of adverse reproductive outcomes (i.e., spontaneous abortions, birth defects, infant mortality) similar in the reclaimed water and control areas? Information on reproductive outcomes would fill a gap in the spectrum of health outcomes included in this assessment.

Monitoring the health of people receiving some reclaimed water in their household water supplies started with the 1984 Health Effects Study, of which epidemiologic studies were an integral part (Nellor et al., 1984, Frerichs et al., 1981, 1982, 1983). Ongoing health surveillance will continue to be an essential part of a program designed to assure the public of the safety of water reclamation.

METHODS USED TO ESTIMATE THE PERCENTAGE OF RECLAIMED WATER IN MONTEBELLO FOREBAY GROUNDWATER SUPPLIES

The following description of the four methods used to estimate the percentage of reclaimed water in the Montebello Forebay groundwater supplies is taken from the report by Bookman-Edmonston Engineering, Inc. (1993a).

SULFATE ION MODELING

The first method used to estimate reclaimed water in the groundwater supply was sulfate ion modeling, a method that uses the sulfate ion as a tracer for groundwater movement. The theory behind this method is that the sulfate concentration in the Colorado River water (a water source used since 1954 to replenish the Montebello Forebay groundwater basin) is substantially higher than the sulfate concentrations of the other types of water in the groundwater basin: stormwater, native groundwater, and reclaimed water. Sulfate is considered a conservative material, the concentration of which is not likely to be affected by either vertical or horizontal movement through soil. Therefore, the sulfate concentration in groundwater pumped from the Montebello Forebay basin was used to estimate the relative proportion of Colorado River water in the groundwater. Any increase in the sulfate concentration at a particular location is indicative of the increased presence of Colorado River water.

In contrast, reclaimed water is not as easily identifiable because of its heterogeneous minerals composition. Because both waters are recharged in the same spreading basins, the relative proportion of reclaimed water in water pumped from a given service area in the groundwater basin can be estimated for any given year from the percentage of Colorado River water derived from sulfate measurements. This method assumes that both types of water follow a similar movement pattern in the groundwater basin. An empirical model was used to derive Colorado River "replacement values," which represent the percentage of native groundwater that has been replaced with Colorado River water through the process of replenishment. The replacement value for a given well in a given year can be calculated using the following equation:

$$R_c = \frac{1}{x} \times \frac{\left(W_s - G_s\right)}{\left(C_s - G_s\right)} \times 100 \quad ,$$

where R_c = percentage replacement of native groundwater with Colorado River water,

$\quad\quad\quad$ W_s = sulfate concentration of a well

$\quad\quad\quad$ G_s = sulfate concentration of native groundwater (assumed constant)

$\quad\quad\quad$ C_s = sulfate concentration of Colorado River water (assumed constant)

$\quad\quad\quad$ x   = dilution factor.

The dilution factor represents the percentage of Colorado River water in the water used to recharge the Montebello Forebay in any given year. Annual dilution factors were calculated for the years 1954 to 1974 and were found not to affect the percentage replacement values significantly. Replacement values for reclaimed water were obtained by shifting replacement values for sulfate by eight years. The eight-year time lag accounts for the difference between the year Colorado River water was first spread (1954) and the year reclaimed water was first spread (1962). The method assumes that the flow of reclaimed water follows the same groundwater dynamics as the flow of Colorado River water, lagged by eight years. This procedure can be represented as

$$R_r\left(1962\right) = R_c\left(1954\right),$$

where R_r = percentage replacement for reclaimed water,

$\quad\quad\quad$ R_c = percentage replacement for Colorado River water.

Finally, the replacement value for reclaimed water was multiplied by the proportional factor F to account for the percentage of reclaimed water in the water used to recharge the basin. Proportional factors were also shifted to account for a time lag between spreading and arrival of reclaimed water at a particular well. Assuming that it takes one year for reclaimed water to reach a particular well, the corresponding proportional factor (F) would be shifted by one year. For example,

$$R_r'\left(1963\right) = R_r\left(1963\right) \times F\left(1962\right) \ .$$

These time values were determined on the basis of the lag between the first spreading of Colorado River water for recharge and the first appearance of sulfate in a particular well. The proportion of reclaimed water in the groundwater supply of a service area is then calculated by summing the volume of reclaimed water in all wells in a service area and dividing it by the total volume of water in a service area. For example, for 1963:

$$P_r\left(1963\right) = \frac{\Sigma\left[R_{ri}\left(1963\right) \times AFY_i\left(1963\right)\right]}{\Sigma \ AFY_i\left(1963\right)} \ ,$$

where P_r =   percentage water pumped that is reclaimed

$\quad\quad\quad$ R_{ri} =   replacement value for reclaimed water for i*th* well,

$\quad\quad\quad$ AFY_i =   total water production for i*th* well.

The sulfate modeling technique could not be used after 1982, because the use of Colorado River water for groundwater recharge in the Montebello Forebay ended in 1974. Because of the eight-year time lag between the spreading of Colorado River water and reclaimed water, Colorado River water replacement values for the years preceding 1974 could be used to determine reclaimed water replacement values, and the percentages of reclaimed water in groundwater, up until 1982. However, after 1982 the sulfate model was used only to a very limited extent. Instead, one of three other analytical methods was employed to derive the annual percentage of reclaimed water in the Montebello Forebay groundwater supplies for the years from 1983 to 1991.

Eventually, the process of groundwater recharge completely replaces the native groundwater. For those wells with 100 percent groundwater replacement prior to 1974, the proportion of reclaimed water in groundwater in any given year was assumed to be equal to the proportion of reclaimed water in the recharge sources X years earlier, where X is the lag time for that well.

REGRESSION ANALYSIS

For the period 1983 to 1991, regression analysis was used to estimate the percentage of reclaimed water for most of the water systems. Using regression methods, the volume of reclaimed water in the groundwater was correlated with the volume of reclaimed water spread based on annual data for 1960 to 1982. If a correlation of 0.80 or greater was found between the volume of reclaimed water in groundwater and the volume of reclaimed water spread in any given year, the regression model was used to predict the percentage of reclaimed water for the water systems for the years 1983 to 1990. If the correlation from the regression was less than 0.80, one of the two remaining techniques was used to estimate the annual percentage of reclaimed water in the groundwater supply.

KRIGING METHOD

For water systems with a correlation of less than 0.80 in the regression analysis, the statistical Kriging technique was used to estimate the percentage of reclaimed water. The Kriging technique assumes that spatial proximity will lead to a high correlation of some parameters. In this case, the assumption was that spatial proximity of two wells would lead to a high correlation between the percentages of reclaimed water in the pumped groundwater from the two wells. Based on this assumption, Bookman-Edmonston Engineering, Inc. used data from wells for which the reclaimed water percentage was known to estimate the percentage of reclaimed water in groundwater pumped from neighboring wells.

TRAVEL TIME CONTOUR METHOD

The travel time contour method was employed to estimate the time required for water to travel from the spreading basin to a particular well in the Montebello Forebay (i.e., "travel time"). This method was used for water systems that had a correlation of less than 0.80 in the regression analysis, and were located too far from another well to use the Kriging technique. It was also used for those few instances when the results from the sulfate-ion method provided clearly erroneous results. It is believed these occurred because of higher-than-normal background sulfate levels, which indicated the arrival of Colorado River recharge water when, in fact, none had yet reached the well in question. This method entailed using a map of the Montebello Forebay showing travel time contours for wells for which this information was known. From these maps, the travel time could be estimated for wells in the region with unknown travel times. The travel time was then used to estimate the percentage of reclaimed water in the groundwater supply using values for wells on the same contour.

ANNUAL PERCENTAGES OF RECLAIMED WATER

Table A.1 (on the following pages) shows estimated annual percentages of reclaimed water for each of the service areas in the Montebello Forebay region. These numbers are the final results of the calculations performed by the staff of Bookman-Edmonston Engineering, Inc. The percentages in Table A.1 are listed by water system number corresponding to the water systems listed below. The letters A, B, C, etc., following the system number in Table A.1 denote service areas within the water system. These service areas are shown on the water system map of the Montebello Forebay (available upon request).

Water System No.	Name of Water System
1	California Water Service Company
3	City of Downey
6	La Habra Heights County Water District
7	Mutual Water Owners Association of Los Nietos
8	City of Montebello
9	Montebello Land and Water Company
10	City of Norwalk
11	Orchard Dale County Water District
12	Park Water Company (part)
13	Pico County Water District
14	City of Pico Rivera
15	San Gabriel Valley Water Company
16	City of Santa Fe Springs
17	South Montebello Irrigation District
18	Southern California Water Company
19	Southwest Suburban Water Company
20	City of Whittier
24	City of Lynwood
25	Maywood Mutual Water Company No. 3
26	Peerless Land and Water Company (part)
28	Rancho Los Amigos
30	City of South Gate
31	Tract No. 180 Mutual Water Company
32	Tract No. 349 Mutual Water Company
33	Bellflower-Somerset Mutual Water Company
34	City of Huntington Park
35	City of Paramount

Table A.1

Estimated Annual Percentage of Reclaimed Water for Montebello Forebay Water System Service Areas

YEAR	1A	1B	1C	1D	3A	3B	3C	3D	3E	3F	6	7	8A	8B	9	10A	10B	10C	10D	11A	11B
1960	0	0	0	0	0	0	0	0	0	0	0	0	0	0	0	0	0	0	0	0	0
1961	0	0	0	0	0	0	0	0	0	0	0	0	0	0	0	0	0	0	0	0	0
1962	0	0	0	0	0	0	0	0	0	0	<1	<1	0	0	0	0	0	0	0	0	0
1963	0	0	0	0	0	0	0	2	0	0	3	3	2	0	0	0	1	0	0	2	0
1964	0	0	0	0	1	0	0	2	2	1	4	4	2	0	0	1	1	0	0	3	0
1965	0	0	0	0	1	0	0	2	2	1	5	5	3	0	2	1	2	0	0	4	0
1966	0	0	0	0	2	<1	0	4	2	1	6	5	3	0	3	1	2	0	0	3	0
1967	0	0	0	0	2	0	1	6	3	2	6	6	4	0	3	2	4	0	0	4	0
1968	0	0	0	0	4	<1	1	10	3	4	10	10	7	0	3	7	7	0	0	8	0
1969	0	0	0	0	5	<1	1	8	6	4	7	8	6	0	4	6	4	1	0	6	0
1970	0	1	0	0	10	<1	1	13	4	5	12	16	9	0	8	6	10	1	0	10	0
1971	0	1	0	1	11	<1	1	15	5	6	14	17	11	0	6	7	12	2	0	9	0
1972	0	1	0	1	14	2	2	22	7	9	21	23	16	0	11	9	12	2	0	18	0
1973	0	1	0	1	13	1	3	15	16	10	15	15	12	0	13	6	8	3	0	15	0
1974	0	1	0	1	17	2	6	17	10	9	15	15	14	0	19	5	7	5	0	12	0
1975	0	2	0	1	14	2	5	17	15	11	17	17	17	0	13	8	8	4	0	17	0
1976	0	3	0	1	18	6	8	22	14	14	23	23	23	0	13	12	11	7	0	20	0
1977	0	0	1	2	18	13	9	13	12	12	21	21	<1	0	15	14	13	0	0	9	9
1978	0	1	1	1	14	10	12	14	11	12	8	9	<1	0	20	10	18	8	0	3	3
1979	0	1	2	2	17	13	15	21	10	14	4	14	9	0	17	14	19	5	0	10	10
1980	0	1	1	3	14	14	20	21	10	19	10	15	14	0	12	12	16	5	0	11	11
1981	0	2	1	4	17	18	18	20	15	17	19	19	19	0	15	14	12	5	0	14	14
1982	0	2	0	2	15	20	9	21	17	8	5	21	0	0	14	18	11	6	0	6	6
1983	0	1	1	3	15	10	14	19	13	12	6	9	0	0	15	14	10	12	0	4	4
1984	0	1	1	2	19	15	11	20	15	10	20	21	0	0	14	21	11	8	0	13	13
1985	0	2	<1	5	12	14	14	21	11	13	14	20	0	0	15	20	9	15	0	10	10
1986	0	1	1	6	16	10	14	20	15	14	13	17	0	0	15	17	8	13	0	7	7
1987	0	1	1	3	19	13	16	19	11	0	21	25	0	0	16	25	9	12	0	12	12
1988	0	1	2	6	20	15	16	17	11	20	21	30	0	0	18	30	10	17	0	17	17
1989	0	0	1	4	22	13	8	16	20	21	18	29	0	0	19	29	10	13	0	10	10
1990	0	0	2	6	26	25	12	16	19	24	27	31	0	0	19	31	11	13	0	17	17
1991	0	0	2	6	26	25	12	16	19	24	27	31	0	0	19	31	11	13	0	17	17

Table A.1—continued

YEAR	12A	12B	12C	12D	12E	12F	12G	12I	13	14A	14B	14C	14D	15A	15B	15C	15D	16	17	18A	18C
1960	0	0	0	0	0	0	0	0	0	0	0	0	0	0	0	0	0	0	0	0	0
1961	0	0	0	0	0	0	0	0	0	0	0	0	0	0	0	0	0	0	0	0	0
1962	0	0	0	0	0	0	0	0	1	0	0	0	0	0	0	5	4	0	0	0	0
1963	0	0	0	0	0	0	0	0	2	1	2	2	<1	0	2	6	5	1	4	0	0
1964	<1	0	0	0	0	0	0	0	3	1	2	2	2	0	3	5	5	2	5	0	0
1965	<1	0	0	0	0	0	0	0	4	2	3	2	2	0	0	6	5	2	5	0	0
1966	<1	0	0	0	0	0	0	0	4	3	4	2	2	0	0	7	6	2	6	0	0
1967	<1	0	0	0	0	0	0	0	5	5	5	2	3	0	0	12	10	4	8	<1	0
1968	<1	0	0	0	0	0	0	0	7	9	8	3	5	0	0	9	9	7	13	1	1
1969	1	0	0	1	0	0	0	0	6	5	8	2	6	0	0	0	12	4	10	1	1
1970	1	0	0	2	0	0	0	0	10	2	14	3	6	0	0	0	15	10	16	2	2
1971	3	0	0	4	0	0	0	0	12	1	6	4	8	0	0	0	20	12	17	2	2
1972	6	0	<1	6	0	0	1	1	17	<1	<1	5	10	0	0	0	16	12	23	2	2
1973	10	0	<1	12	0	<1	<1	1	15	1	1	6	17	0	0	0	15	8	15	1	8
1974	9	0	<1	14	0	<1	1	1	16	2	1	4	12	0	0	0	17	7	15	1	8
1975	8	0	0	14	0	<1	1	1	16	<1	1	9	16	0	0	0	22	8	17	1	9
1976	11	0	<1	20	0	0	1	3	15	21	13	13	16	0	11	0	20	11	23	1	9
1977	0	23	0	22	0	0	3	5	15	9	18	13	15	0	2	0	23	13	21	5	8
1978	0	2	0	9	0	0	6	7	16	14	14	6	14	0	0	0	23	18	9	6	8
1979	0	7	0	13	<1	0	7	4	14	15	16	7	0	0	0	0	25	19	14	5	12
1980	0	0	<1	14	<1	0	4	4	17	17	11	5	0	0	0	0	22	16	15	5	12
1981	0	0	<1	18	1	0	6	3	16	18	15	7	0	0	0	0	23	12	19	6	12
1982	0	10	1	20	<1	0	9	2	20	9	16	8	0	0	0	0	19	11	21	9	13
1983	0	4	1	9	1	0	11	4	17	21	13	6	0	0	0	0	23	10	9	7	9
1984	0	5	1	16	1	0	9	<1	19	20	20	12	0	0	0	0	21	11	21	6	6
1985	0	5	1	15	1	0	1	0	16	17	21	8	0	0	0	0	23	9	20	6	6
1986	0	9	2	12	<1	0	0	1	18	25	20	8	0	0	0	0	24	8	17	8	5
1987	0	0	2	18	1	0	1	1	20	30	22	12	0	0	0	0	29	9	25	7	8
1988	0	0	3	22	2	0	2	2	16	29	26	15	0	0	0	0	26	10	30	11	9
1989	0	19	4	21	2	0	2	3	17	31	27	11	0	0	0	0	30	10	29	9	12
1990	0	0	4	28	2	0	6	3	14	31	29	27	0	0	0	0	30	11	31	12	15
1991	0	0	4	28	2	0	6	3	14	31	29	27	0	0	0	0	30	11	31	12	15

Table A.1—continued

YEAR	18D	18E	18F	18G	19A	19B	20	24	25	26A	26B	26C	26D	28	30A	30B	31	32	33	34	35
1960	0	0	0	0	0	0	0	0	0	0	0	0	0	0	0	0	0	0	—	—	—
1961	0	0	0	0	0	0	0	0	0	0	0	0	0	0	0	0	0	0	—	—	—
1962	0	0	0	0	0	0	<1	0	0	0	0	0	0	0	0	0	0	0	—	—	—
1963	0	0	0	0	0	0	0	0	0	0	0	0	0	0	0	0	0	0	—	—	—
1964	0	0	0	0	0	0	0	0	0	0	0	0	0	0	0	0	0	0	—	—	—
1965	0	0	0	0	0	0	0	0	0	0	0	0	0	0	0	0	0	0	—	—	—
1966	0	0	0	0	0	0	0	0	0	0	0	0	0	0	0	0	0	0	—	—	—
1967	0	<1	1	<1	0	0	0	0	0	0	0	0	0	0	0	0	0	0	—	—	—
1968	0	<1	1	<1	0	0	0	0	0	0	0	0	0	0	0	0	0	0	—	—	—
1969	0	<1	1	<1	0	0	0	0	0	0	0	1	0	0	0	1	0	0	—	—	—
1970	0	<1	1	<1	0	0	0	0	0	0	0	1	0	<1	1	2	0	0	—	—	—
1971	0	<1	1	<1	0	0	0	0	0	0	0	2	0	<1	1	2	0	0	—	—	—
1972	0	1	2	1	0	0	0	0	0	0	0	2	0	2	1	3	0	0	—	—	—
1973	0	1	2	2	0	0	0	<1	0	0	0	2	0	2	1	3	0	0	—	—	—
1974	0	<1	4	3	0	0	0	<1	0	2	1	4	0	4	3	6	0	0	—	—	—
1975	0	<1	4	4	0	0	<1	<1	0	3	2	3	<1	3	4	5	0	0	—	—	—
1976	0	<1	5	15	0	0	0	<1	0	3	3	4	<1	9	3	23	0	0	0	0	0
1977	<1	4	5	9	0	0	0	1	1	9	3	5	<1	1	2	2	0	0	0	0	0
1978	0	4	10	13	0	0	0	2	1	12	9	5	<1	13	1	7	0	0	0	0	0
1979	0	7	11	14	0	0	0	1	1	13	10	6	1	5	1	0	0	0	0	2	0
1980	0	9	17	18	0	0	0	1	2	15	11	5	1	7	1	0	0	0	0	2	<1
1981	0	13	22	20	0	0	0	1	2	15	13	5	1	12	1	10	0	0	0	2	<1
1982	<1	13	22	9	0	0	0	1	3	17	15	4	1	14	1	4	0	0	0	2	1
1983	0	17	20	16	0	0	0	0	1	15	17	4	1	10	0	5	0	0	1	1	1
1984	0	14	23	15	0	0	0	<1	2	16	16	2	2	8	3	5	0	0	1	1	1
1985	0	19	24	12	0	0	0	0	2	15	16	1	3	10	7	9	0	0	1	2	1
1986	0	18	27	18	0	0	<1	0	2	14	17	1	4	10	7	0	0	0	1	1	2
1987	0	20	26	22	0	0	<1	0	2	15	14	0	2	8	9	0	0	0	2	1	2
1988	0	22	20	21	0	0	0	<1	1	19	15	0	3	12	9	19	0	0	2	1	3
1989	0	17	23	28	0	0	0	<1	2	21	19	0	4	13	9	0	0	0	2	1	4
1990	0	21	23	28	0	0	0	<1	2	19	21	0	4	12	9	0	0	0	2	2	4
1991	0	21	23	28	0	0	0	<1	2	19	19	0	4	12	9	0	0	0	2	2	4

1990 CENSUS TRACTS IN FIVE EXPOSURE AREAS USED IN THE ANALYSES OF CANCER INCIDENCE AND MORTALITY DATA

		RW 1		
4827.00	5020.02	5326.01	5401.01	5540.00
5013.00	5030.00	5326.02	5401.02	5541.00
5014.00	5309.00	5327.00	5402.00	5544.01
5015.01	5310.00	5330.00	5403.00	5544.02
5015.02	5315.02	5331.01	5405.00	5548.01
5016.00	5316.02	5331.02	5417.00	
5017.00	5317.02	5332.00	5533.00	
5018.00	5323.02	5345.00	5537.00	
5019.00	5325.00	5400.00	5538.00	
		RW 2		
5012.00	5302.02	5312.02	5318.00	5532.00
5029.01	5303.00	5313.01	5319.01	5535.00
5031.01	5304.00	5313.02	5319.02	5536.00
5031.02	5305.00	5315.01	5340.00	5547.00
5033.02	5311.00	5316.01	5527.00	
5300.02	5312.01	5317.01	5531.00	
		RW 3		
4087.01	5338.02	5356.02	5361.00	5522.00
5021.00	5339.00	5357.00	5362.00	5523.00
5035.01	5341.00	5358.01	5503.00	5528.00
5300.01	5342.00	5358.02	5504.00	5529.00
5302.01	5355.00	5359.00	5519.00	5530.00
5338.01	5356.01	5360.00	5520.00	5546.00
		RW 4		
5002.01	5032.02	5508.00	5513.00	5518.00
5025.00	5336.00	5509.00	5514.00	5521.00
5026.01	5500.00	5510.00	5515.00	5534.00
5026.02	5501.00	5511.00	5516.00	
5032.01	5502.00	5512.00	5517.00	
		RW 5		
5001.00	5006.00	5010.00	5301.01	5505.00
5004.01	5007.00	5022.00	5301.02	5506.00
5004.02	5008.00	5023.00	5320.00	5507.00
5005.00	5009.00	5024.00	5321.00	

1990 CENSUS TRACTS IN FIVE RECLAIMED WATER AREAS USED IN THE ANALYSES OF INFECTIOUS DISEASE DATA

		RW 1		
4827.00	5317.02	5330.00	5401.01	5519.00
5029.01	5323.02	5331.01	5401.02	5533.00
5031.02	5325.00	5331.02	5402.00	5540.00
5309.00	5326.01	5332.00	5403.00	5544.01
5315.02	5326.02	5345.00	5405.00	5548.01
5316.02	5327.00	5400.00	5417.00	

		RW 2		
5012.00	5304.00	5313.01	5520.00	5541.00
5031.01	5305.00	5313.02	5527.00	5544.02
5033.02	5310.00	5315.01	5531.00	5547.00
5300.01	5311.00	5316.01	5532.00	
5300.02	5312.01	5317.01	5537.00	
5303.00	5312.02	5340.00	5538.00	

		RW 3		
4087.01	5318.00	5356.01	5360.00	5528.00
5002.01	5319.01	5356.02	5361.00	5529.00
5021.00	5319.02	5357.00	5362.00	5530.00
5035.01	5339.00	5358.01	5504.00	5535.00
5302.01	5341.00	5358.02	5522.00	5536.00
5302.02	5355.00	5359.00	5523.00	5546.00

		RW 4		
5032.01	5338.01	5502.00	5511.00	5516.00
5032.02	5338.02	5503.00	5512.00	5517.00
5301.01	5342.00	5508.00	5513.00	5518.00
5301.02	5500.00	5509.00	5514.00	5521.00
5321.00	5501.00	5510.00	5515.00	5534.00

		RW 5		
5001.00	5006.00	5010.00	5025.00	5336.00
5004.01	5007.00	5022.00	5026.01	5505.00
5004.02	5008.00	5023.00	5026.02	5506.00
5005.00	5009.00	5024.00	5320.00	5507.00

1990 CENSUS TRACTS IN CONTROL AREA USED IN THE ANALYSES OF ALL HEALTH OUTCOMES DATA

		Montebello Forebay Control		
5002.02	5034.01	5036.01	5343.00	
5020.01	5034.02	5036.02	5344.01	
5033.01	5035.02	5037.01	5344.02	

		Pomona Control		
4017.02	4023.02	4025.02	4029.01	4088.00
4021.01	4024.01	4026.00	4029.02	
4021.02	4024.02	4027.01	4030.00	
4022.00	4024.03	4027.02	4032.00	
4023.01	4025.01	4028.00	4033.11	

		San Fernando Valley Control		
1044.01	1070.00	1190.00	1216.00	1237.00
1044.02	1091.00	1191.00	1218.00	1238.00
1045.00	1092.00	1192.00	1219.00	1239.00
1046.00	1093.00	1193.00	1220.00	1271.01
1047.01	1094.00	1194.00	1221.00	1271.02
1047.02	1095.00	1197.00	1222.00	1272.00
1048.00	1096.01	1198.00	1224.00	1273.00
1060.00	1096.02	1199.00	1230.00	1274.00
1061.02	1171.00	1200.00	1232.01	1276.01
1061.11	1172.00	1201.01	1232.02	1276.02
1061.12	1173.01	1201.02	1233.01	1277.00
1064.01	1173.02	1203.00	1233.02	1278.01
1064.02	1173.03	1204.00	1234.00	1278.02
1065.00	1174.01	1210.00	1235.00	1279.00
1066.01	1174.04	1211.00	1236.01	3201.00
1066.02	1175.00	1212.00	1236.02	3202.00
				3203.00

CHARACTERISTICS OF POPULATIONS LIVING IN ANALYSIS SUBAREAS WITHIN RECLAIMED WATER AND CONTROL AREAS

Table E.1

Characteristics of Populations Living in Reclaimed Water Areas Used in Cancer and Mortality Analyses

Characteristic (in 1990)	Area				
	RW 1	RW 2	RW 3	RW 4	RW 5
Population	260,131	171,889	226,094	133,978	116,129
	Percent				
Hispanic	66.2	73.5	68.2	45.1	69.9
Non-Hispanic					
White	22.7	17.5	23.1	44.6	25.1
Black	6.3	2.2	1.9	2.7	5.3
Asian	4.2	6.2	6.3	6.8	3.9
Persons 0–17 years	32.4	32.5	32.9	27.2	28.6
Persons 65 years and older	8.1	8.0	7.6	11.0	11.5
Persons who are not U.S. citizens	31.6	30.6	32.4	20.3	21.0
Families below poverty level	15.2	14.5	13.1	7.9	8.9
Employed in white-collar occupations	15.1	14.8	14.6	20.6	18.9
Adults with eight years of education or less	29.5	30.2	27.7	14.3	19.4
Adults with high school education or more	50.8	48.0	52.3	68.5	58.9
Housing units that are renter-occupied	58.4	51.4	50.2	46.7	34.8
Living in same house for at least 5 years	48.0	55.5	47.2	50.4	58.9
Moved into current residence in 1989–1990	24.0	20.8	23.8	22.7	15.5

Table E.2

**Characteristics of Populations Living in Reclaimed Water Areas Used
in Infectious Disease Analyses**

Characteristic (in 1990)	Area				
	RW 1	RW 2	RW 3	RW 4	RW 5
Population	180,017	177,787	212,903	154,903	127,827
			Percent		
Hispanic	73.7	67.8	68.1	50.4	71.9
Non-Hispanic					
White	14.5	21.5	22.6	39.7	23.4
Black	7.1	2.5	2.9	2.5	0.5
Asian	4.1	7.3	5.8	6.5	3.5
Persons 0–17 years	33.7	31.9	32.8	28.6	29.4
Persons 65 years and older	7.2	8.3	7.8	10.6	10.3
Persons who are not U.S. citizens	35.6	29.9	31.3	24.1	23.2
Families below poverty level	17.2	14.2	12.7	9.6	10.2
Employed in white-collar occupations	12.2	15.5	15.3	18.3	17.8
Adults with eight years of education or less	35.3	28.6	27.4	17.2	21.5
Adults with high school education or more	43.2	50.7	52.7	63.8	57.2
Housing units that are renter-occupied	55.6	54.1	49.3	52.3	34.9
Living in same house for at least 5 years	51.5	53.5	47.6	48.7	57.7
Moved into current residence in 1989–1990	21.3	22.2	23.7	24.1	16.1

Table E.3

Characteristics of Populations Living in the Control Area, Based on the 1990 U.S. Census

Characteristic (in 1990)	Montebello Forebay Control	Pomona Control	San Fernando Valley Control
Population	80,082	136,711	457,278
	Percent		
Hispanic	58.3	49.3	52.2
Non-Hispanic			
White	35.4	29.4	34.9
Black	2.3	13.7	4.4
Asian	3.3	7.1	7.9
Persons 0–17 years	29.1	32.7	28.7
Persons 65 years and older	9.0	6.4	8.0
Persons who are not U.S. citizens	26.2	24.8	31.8
Families below poverty level	11.1	13.2	11.3
Employed in white-collar occupations	19.5	21.0	19.5
Adults with eight years of education or less	21.5	20.7	21.5
Adults with high school education or more	60.8	61.2	60.9
Housing units that are renter-occupied	42.5	41.0	49.5
Living in same house for at least 5 years	54.1	40.0	44.7
Moved into current residence in 1989–1990	17.6	28.0	25.3

NUMBER OF CANCERS, DEATHS, AND CASES OF INFECTIOUS DISEASE OCCURRING IN THE RECLAIMED WATER AREAS AND CONTROL AREA

Table F.1

Number of Incident Cases of Cancer by Site in the Reclaimed Water and Control Areas, 1987–1991

Cancer Site	Area					
	RW 1	RW 2	RW 3	RW 4	RW 5	Control
All sites	3864	2468	3298	2725	2142	10607
Bladder	142	87	125	108	97	452
Colon	327	184	263	257	178	852
Esophagus	32	20	26	24	20	77
Kidney	58	48	60	42	42	192
Liver	34	33	25	23	34	87
Pancreas	93	58	91	56	54	238
Rectum	90	44	77	70	48	237
Stomach	110	91	99	71	53	274

Table F.2

Number of Deaths by Cause in the Reclaimed Water and Control Areas, 1989–1991

Cause of Death	Area					
	RW 1	RW 2	RW 3	RW 4	RW 5	Control
All causes	4250	2763	3560	2630	2288	10894
Cancer						
All sites	840	559	761	601	530	2262
Bladder	15	7	10	9	7	35
Colon	67	47	71	48	32	192
Esophagus	20	8	9	15	7	44
Kidney	16	17	9	9	6	50
Liver	26	19	19	14	20	63
Pancreas	44	30	40	28	31	117
Rectum	8	8	8	5	7	21
Stomach	39	39	36	31	29	80
Heart disease	1466	924	1256	950	815	3820
Cerebrovascular disease	288	148	227	157	136	638
All other	1656	1132	1316	922	807	4174

Table F.3

Number of Cases of Selected Infectious Diseases in the Reclaimed Water and Control Areas, 1989–1990

Disease	Area					
	RW 1	RW 2	RW 3	RW 4	RW 5	Control
Giardia	75	95	65	38	31	228
Hepatitis A	80	93	110	56	52	225
Salmonella	60	74	69	59	36	225
Shigella	128	107	127	60	64	273
Other [a]	35	31	31	18	27	105
All of the above	378	400	402	231	210	1056

[a]Includes typhoid fever, amebiasis, unspecified meningitis, leptospirosis, cholera, and gastroenteritis.

RESULTS OF SENSITIVITY ANALYSES FOR CANCER INCIDENCE

RESULTS CONTROLLING FOR AGE AND SEX

The cancer results based on models that control only for age and sex (Table G.1) show patterns similar to those described in Chapter Four. In general, the rate ratios are somewhat smaller in magnitude than those generated by the analyses adjusting for age, sex, and ethnicity. Because the lower rates of cancer among Hispanics (observed in our data) are not taken into account in these results, the rates in the reclaimed water areas (with more Hispanics) are lower than the rates in the control areas (with slightly fewer Hispanics). The rank order (i.e., from lowest to highest) of the rate ratios representing the five reclaimed water areas is similar between the two analyses (Table 4.2 and Table G.1) for kidney, liver, pancreas, rectum, and stomach cancer. Notably, in Table G.1, the RW 2 area has the lowest rate ratios and the RW 4 area has the highest rate ratios for four categories: all sites, bladder, colon, and esophagus, in contrast to the ranks in Table 4.2.

RESULTS CONTROLLING FOR AGE, SEX, ETHNICITY, AND INCOME

The model controlling for age, sex, ethnicity, and income yielded a pattern of cancer results (Table G.2) almost identical with those from the model controlling for age, sex, and ethnicity (Table 4.2). In models for five of the nine cancers, the income variable was not significant (results not shown). The rate ratios from the model controlling for income are slightly lower for RW 1, RW 2, and RW 3 and slightly higher for RW 4 and RW 5, indicating that people with similar incomes have slightly lower rates in RW 1, RW 2, and RW 3, and slightly higher rates in RW 4 and RW 5. Although there are a few differences in the rank order of the rate ratios representing the five reclaimed water areas, generally the patterns are the same.

Table G.1

Rate Ratios and Confidence Intervals for Cancer Incidence, Controlling for Age and Sex, 1987–1991

Cancer site	Area					
	RW 1	RW 2	RW 3	RW 4	RW 5	Control
All sites	0.96 (0.90–1.02)	0.90[a] (0.83–0.98)	0.95 (0.89–1.01)	1.01 (0.95–1.07)	0.90[a] (0.84–0.97)	1.00
Bladder	0.83 (0.65–1.05)	0.74[a] (0.56–0.99)	0.86 (0.72–1.04)	0.89 (0.72–1.09)	0.88 (0.68–1.15)	1.00
Colon	0.99 (0.85–1.15)	0.82[a] (0.72–0.93)	0.94 (0.83–1.07)	1.12 (0.93–1.35)	0.87 (0.75–1.01)	1.00
Esophagus	1.13 (0.75–1.71)	1.01 (0.64–1.60)	1.06 (0.59–1.91)	1.18 (0.84–1.66)	1.10 (0.65–1.85)	1.00
Kidney	0.82 (0.58–1.16)	0.98 (0.72–1.33)	0.97 (0.74–1.28)	0.87 (0.63–1.20)	0.98 (0.69–1.40)	1.00
Liver	0.99 (0.61–1.61)	1.44 (0.93–2.23)	0.89 (0.55–1.45)	1.04 (0.71–1.53)	1.73[a] (1.11–2.70)	1.00
Pancreas	1.03 (0.81–1.32)	0.95 (0.71–1.26)	1.17 (0.91–1.51)	0.89 (0.69–1.14)	0.96 (0.70–1.31)	1.00
Rectum	0.99 (0.77–1.29)	0.72[a] (0.53–0.97)	1.00 (0.79–1.27)	1.11 (0.85–1.45)	0.85 (0.61–1.19)	1.00
Stomach	1.06 (0.83–1.34)	1.27[a] (1.01–1.60)	1.11 (0.91–1.36)	0.99 (0.79–1.24)	0.83 (0.64–1.09)	1.00

[a]Statistically significantly different from 1.0 (p > 0.05).

Table G.2

Rate Ratios and Confidence Intervals for Cancer Incidence, Controlling for Age, Sex, Ethnicity, and Income, 1987–1991

Cancer site	Area					
	RW 1	RW 2	RW 3	RW 4	RW 5	Control
All sites	1.03 (0.98–1.08)	1.10[a] (1.03–1.19)	1.02 (0.96–1.09)	1.00 (0.96–1.05)	1.05 (0.99–1.12)	1.00
Bladder	0.93 (0.75–1.15)	1.00 (0.78–1.28)	0.94 (0.79–1.11)	0.86 (0.69–1.08)	1.04 (0.81–1.33)	1.00
Colon	1.06 (0.93–1.21)	1.06 (0.92–1.22)	1.03 (0.90–1.17)	1.14 (0.96–1.35)	1.04 (0.91–1.20)	1.00
Esophagus	1.06 (0.71–1.58)	1.17 (0.73–1.89)	1.09 (0.62–1.93)	1.33 (0.91–1.94)	1.42 (0.82–2.44)	1.00
Kidney	0.82 (0.58–1.16)	1.08 (0.78–1.48)	1.01 (0.77–1.34)	0.88 (0.64–1.21)	1.05 (0.74–1.49)	1.00
Liver	0.97 (0.60–1.55)	1.34 (0.85–2.12)	0.87 (0.53–1.42)	1.04 (0.71–1.52)	1.76[a] (1.11–2.79)	1.00
Pancreas	1.06 (0.84–1.33)	1.09 (0.80–1.48)	1.23 (0.95–1.58)	0.90 (0.70–1.16)	1.07 (0.77–1.49)	1.00
Rectum	1.06 (0.82–1.37)	0.87 (0.64–1.18)	1.07 (0.85–1.35)	1.11 (0.85–1.45)	0.98 (0.70–1.38)	1.00
Stomach	1.04 (0.82–1.32)	1.25 (0.99–1.59)	1.10 (0.89–1.35)	1.02 (0.82–1.28)	0.87 (0.66–1.15)	1.00

[a]Statistically significantly different from 1.0 (p < 0.05).

RESULTS OF SENSITIVITY ANALYSES FOR MORTALITY

RESULTS CONTROLLING FOR AGE AND SEX

Generally, the rate ratios for mortality from the model controlling for age and sex (Table H.1) are slightly smaller in magnitude than those from the model that also controls for ethnicity (Table 4.3). The rate ratios for stomach cancer, however, are slightly larger, probably resulting from a higher death rate due to stomach cancer among Hispanics. Despite some differences in the rank order of the rate ratios, the conclusion of no relationship between reclaimed water and mortality still holds.

RESULTS CONTROLLING FOR AGE, SEX, ETHNICITY, AND INCOME

The rate ratios based on the model that controls for income in addition to age, sex, and ethnicity (Table H.2) are similar in magnitude to those from the model controlling for age, sex, and ethnicity (Table 4.3). In models for 8 of the 13 causes of death, the income variable was not significant (results not shown). Generally, the rate ratios are slightly smaller for RW 1, RW 2, and RW 3, indicating that people with the same income have slightly lower rates than in the control area. Rate ratios controlling for income are of the same magnitude or slightly larger for RW 4 and RW 5, indicating that people of the same income have similar or higher rates than in the control area.

Table H.1

**Rate Ratios and Confidence Intervals for Mortality, Controlling
for Age and Sex, 1989–1991**

Cause of Death	Area					
	RW 1	RW 2	RW 3	RW 4	RW 5	Control
All causes	0.98 (0.92–1.05)	0.98 (0.89–1.07)	1.00 (0.93–1.07)	0.95 (0.88–1.03)	0.94 (0.87–1.01)	1.00
Cancer						
All sites	0.97 (0.89–1.06)	0.95 (0.84–1.08)	1.03 (0.95–1.12)	1.01 (0.92–1.11)	1.00 (0.90–1.11)	1.00
Bladder	1.08 (0.60–1.96)	0.76 (0.35–1.66)	0.88 (0.48–1.63)	0.95 (0.49–1.88)	0.82 (0.36–1.91)	1.00
Colon	0.88 (0.66–1.18)	0.94 (0.67–1.31)	1.13 (0.83–1.54)	0.93 (0.67–1.30)	0.70 (0.49–1.00)	1.00
Esophagus	1.22 (0.71–2.08)	0.70 (0.29–1.71)	0.64 (0.30–1.35)	1.29 (0.72–2.32)	0.67 (0.22–2.09)	1.00
Kidney	0.85 (0.49–1.47)	1.31 (0.77–2.25)	0.56 (0.27–1.13)	0.68 (0.36–1.27)	0.51 (0.20–1.29)	1.00
Liver	1.07 (0.68–1.71)	1.16 (0.73–1.85)	0.93 (0.61–1.41)	0.84 (0.47–1.51)	1.35 (0.85–2.13)	1.00
Pancreas	0.97 (0.68–1.39)	0.98 (0.63–1.52)	1.05 (0.72–1.52)	0.89 (0.57–1.37)	1.10 (0.76–1.59)	1.00
Rectum	0.98 (0.43–2.21)	1.46 (0.65–3.29)	1.17 (0.49–2.80)	0.87 (0.35–2.20)	1.37 (0.53–3.54)	1.00
Stomach	1.27 (0.82–1.97)	1.87[a] (1.27–2.76)	1.38 (0.92–2.07)	1.46 (0.93–2.30)	1.53[a] (1.01–2.33)	1.00
Heart disease	0.95 (0.86–1.05)	0.93 (0.82–1.04)	1.01 (0.91–1.11)	0.93 (0.84–1.03)	0.90 (0.82–1.00)	1.00
Cerebrovascular disease	1.11 (0.96–1.29)	0.89 (0.73–1.10)	1.08 (0.93–1.26)	0.92 (0.76–1.13)	0.91 (0.75–1.11)	1.00
All other	1.01 (0.93–1.10)	1.05 (0.95–1.17)	0.96 (0.88–1.04)	0.94 (0.85–1.05)	0.94 (0.83–1.06)	1.00

[a]Statistically significantly different from 1.0 ($p < 0.05$).

Table H.2

Rate Ratios and Confidence Intervals for Mortality, Controlling for Age, Sex, Ethnicity, and Income, 1989–1991

Cause of Death	Area					
	RW 1	RW 2	RW 3	RW 4	RW 5	Control
All causes	1.00 (0.92–1.08)	1.15[a] (1.05–1.26)	1.05 (0.98–1.12)	0.98 (0.90–1.06)	1.08 (0.98–1.18)	1.00
Cancer						
All sites	1.03 (0.94–1.12)	1.17[a] (1.02–1.34)	1.10[a] (1.01–1.20)	1.01 (0.92–1.12)	1.16[a] 1.06–1.28)	1.00
Bladder	1.14 (0.62–2.11)	0.98 (0.43–2.25)	0.94 (0.50–1.75)	0.85 (0.43–1.66)	0.95 (0.41–2.24)	1.00
Colon	1.00 (0.76–1.31)	1.32 (0.96–1.82)	1.26 (0.92–1.73)	0.93 (0.67–1.29)	0.86 (0.59–1.26)	1.00
Esophagus	1.24 (0.72–2.12)	0.83 (0.34–2.05)	0.66 (0.31–1.42)	1.33 (0.73–2.40)	0.78 (0.25–2.49)	1.00
Kidney	0.86 (0.48–1.53)	1.36 (0.75–2.48)	0.55 (0.27–1.13)	0.66 (0.35––1.24)	0.51 (0.20–1.28)	1.00
Liver	1.02 (0.65–1.61)	1.14 (0.71–1.83)	0.87 (0.58–1.33)	0.90 (0.50–1.62)	1.46 (0.90–2.35)	1.00
Pancreas	1.02 (0.72–1.44)	1.22 (0.78–1.93)	1.15 (0.79–1.67)	0.90 (0.58–1.40)	1.25 (0.84–1.87)	1.00
Rectum	0.98 (0.45–2.11)	1.65 (0.72–3.79)	1.22 (0.51–2.90)	0.91 (0.35–2.38)	1.54 (0.57–4.11)	1.00
Stomach	1.28 (0.83–1.97)	1.74[a] (1.18–2.57)	1.36 (0.90–2.05)	1.49 (0.95–2.32)	1.48 (0.98–2.23)	1.00
Heart disease	0.97 (0.88–1.07)	1.15[a] (1.03–1.28)	1.07 (0.98–1.17)	0.97 (0.87–1.08)	1.05 (0.93–1.19)	1.00
Cerebrovascular disease	1.12 (0.96–1.30)	1.05 (0.86–1.29)	1.11 (0.95–1.30)	0.95 (0.78–1.18)	1.02 (0.83–1.25)	1.00
All other	0.99 (0.90–1.09)	1.16[a] (1.05–1.29)	1.00 (0.92–1.08)	0.97 (0.87–1.08)	1.07 (0.95–1.22)	1.00

[a]Statistically significantly different from 1.0 ($p < 0.05$).

RESULTS OF SENSITIVITY ANALYSES FOR INFECTIOUS DISEASE INCIDENCE

RESULTS CONTROLLING FOR AGE AND SEX

Almost all the rate ratios for infectious diseases from the model controlling only for age and sex (Table I.1) are slightly larger than those also controlling for ethnicity (Table 4.4). This indicates that Hispanics, whites, and/or the "other" subgroup have higher rates of infectious disease in the reclaimed water areas than the corresponding subgroup in the control area. The magnitude of the rate ratios in relation to the other reclaimed water areas (i.e., rank order) and relative to the control area is about the same in the two analyses, meaning the qualitative conclusions remain unchanged.

RESULTS CONTROLLING FOR AGE, SEX, ETHNICITY, AND INCOME

The rate ratios from the model that controls for income differences in addition to age, sex, and ethnicity (Table I.2) are slightly smaller than those not controlling for income (Table 4.4). In three of the six models, the income variable was not significant (results not shown). The relative magnitude of the five rate ratios for each infectious disease category is similar in the two analyses, indicating that the conclusions drawn from the main analyses describe these results as well.

Table I.1

Rate Ratios and Confidence Intervals for Infectious Disease Incidence, Controlling for Age and Sex, 1989–1990

| Disease | Area | | | | | |
	RW 1	RW 2	RW 3	RW 4	RW 5	Control
Giardia	1.14 (0.78–1.65)	1.55[a] (1.11–2.15)	0.86 (0.60–1.24)	0.76 (0.52–1.12)	0.75 (0.42–1.32)	1.00
Hepatitis A	1.24 (0.93–1.66)	1.52[a] (1.10–2.10)	1.48[a] (1.10–1.98)	1.12 (0.73–1.70)	1.23 (0.90–1.68)	1.00
Salmonella	0.96 (0.74–1.25)	1.25 (0.99–1.57)	0.95 (0.75–1.22)	1.17 (0.86–1.57)	0.87 (0.56–1.33)	1.00
Shigella	1.63[a] (1.30–2.03)	1.46[a] (1.12–1.89)	1.41[a] (1.12–1.77)	1.00 (0.71–1.42)	1.27 (0.90–1.78)	1.00
Other[b]	1.20 (0.78–1.83)	1.10 (0.72–1.67)	0.91 (0.55–1.50)	0.84 (0.47–1.52)	1.37 (0.80–2.35)	1.00
All of the above	1.26[a] (1.05–1.50)	1.41[a] (1.21–1.64)	1.16 (1.00–1.35)	0.99 (0.84–1.18)	1.07 (0.85–1.37)	1.00

[a]Statistically significantly different from 1.0 ($p < 0.05$).
[b]Includes typhoid fever, amebiasis, unspecified meningitis, leptospirosis, cholera, and gastroenteritis.

Table I.2

Rate Ratios and Confidence Intervals for Infectious Disease Incidence, Controlling for Age, Sex, Ethnicity, and Income, 1989–1990

| Disease | Area | | | | | |
	RW 1	RW 2	RW 3	RW 4	RW 5	Control
Giardia	0.94 (0.63–1.41)	1.36 (0.98–1.87)	0.79 (0.55–1.13)	0.76 (0.51–1.14)	0.71 (0.39–1.30)	1.00
Hepatitis A	1.08 (0.80–1.44)	1.38 (0.98–1.94)	1.37[a] (1.04–1.81)	1.11 (0.73–1.68)	1.16 (0.84–1.60)	1.00
Salmonella	0.94 (0.72–1.21)	1.21 (0.95–1.54)	0.93 (0.73–1.19)	1.17 (0.87–1.59)	0.82 (0.53–1.26)	1.00
Shigella	1.36[a] (1.08–1.70)	1.28 (1.00–1.63)	1.27[a] (1.03–1.56)	1.02 (0.75–1.39)	1.14 (0.84–1.55)	1.00
Other[b]	1.14 (0.71–1.85)	1.07 (0.70–1.65)	0.91 (0.55–1.52)	0.77 (0.41–1.48)	1.44 (0.86–2.42)	1.00
All of the above	1.10 (0.91–1.33)	1.28[a] (1.12–1.47)	1.08 (0.94–1.24)	0.99 (0.83–1.18)	1.01 (0.80–1.28)	1.00

[a]Statistically significantly different from 1.0 ($p < 0.05$).
[b]Includes typhoid fever, amebiasis, unspecified meningitis, leptospirosis, cholera, and gastroenteritis.

SUMMARY OF RESULTS OF SENSITIVITY ANALYSES FOR SEPARATE CONTROL AREA LOCATIONS

Census tracts in three Los Angeles County locations were combined and used as a single control area in the analyses in this report: Montebello Forebay (MFB), Pomona, and San Fernando Valley (SFV). To assess the impact on the results of separating the control locations, rates of cancer incidence, mortality, and infectious disease were compared between these three locations and between the three control locations and the reclaimed water areas.

CANCER INCIDENCE

Rates of cancer tend to be higher (but typically not significantly higher) in the SFV control tracts than in the MFB control region. Cancer rates tend to be lower (again, not significantly lower) for the Pomona control region than for the MFB control tracts. The rates in the reclaimed water areas tend not to be significantly different from the MFB control, except for all cancers and all other cancers [not gastrointestanal (GI)]. Also, RW 2 and RW 5 have significantly higher rates of liver cancer than the MFB control and RW 2 has a significantly higher rate of stomach cancer. The reclaimed water areas tend to have higher rates than the Pomona control, although these differences are rarely significant. RW 2 and RW 3 have higher cancer rates than the SFV control area for 10 of the 12 outcomes. RW 1 has higher rates than the SFV control area on eight outcomes and RW 5 has higher rates than the SFV control area on half the outcomes. The rates for RW 4 are typically lower than for the SFV controls. Almost none of these differences are statistically significant, the exceptions being for all cancers and all other (not GI) cancers for which the rates for RW 2 are significantly higher, and the rates for RW 4 are significantly lower than for the SFV control area.

MORTALITY

There are almost no statistically significant differences between the control areas in the death rates for the causes of death analyzed. The only exceptions are that the Pomona control region has a significantly higher rate of death from all causes and death from other causes than does the MFB control area.

INFECTIOUS DISEASE

The Pomona control area has the highest rates of infectious disease. It has significantly higher rates of all infectious diseases, giardia, and hepatitis A than the MFB control area and significantly higher rates of all infectious diseases, hepatitis A, and all other infectious diseases than the SFV control area. The rate of disease is lower in the SFV control area than in the Pomona control area for all outcomes. The Pomona control area also tends to have higher rates of disease than the reclaimed water areas, although the differences are typically not significant. The exception is shigella, for which RW 1, 2, and 3 have slightly but not significantly higher rates of disease.

Alavanja, M., I. Goldstein, and M. Susser, "A Case-Control Study of Gastrointestinal and Urinary Tract Cancer Mortality and Drinking Water Chlorination," in R. L. Jolley, H. Gorchev, D. H. Hamilton, Jr. (eds.), *Water Chlorination: Environmental Impact and Health Effects*, 2nd ed., Ann Arbor, Michigan: Ann Arbor Science Publishers, 1978, pp. 395–409.

Ames, B. N., "Dietary Carcinogens and Anticarcinogens, Oxygen Radicals and Degenerative Diseases," *Science*, Vol. 221, 1983, pp. 1256–1264.

Bean, J. A., P. Isaacson, W. J. Hausler, et al., "Drinking Water and Cancer Incidence in Iowa: I. Trends and Incidence by Source of Drinking Water and Size of Municipality," *American Journal of Epidemiology*, Vol. 116, No. 6, 1982a, pp. 912–923.

Bean, J. A., P. Isaacson, R. M. A. Hahne, et al., "Drinking Water and Cancer Incidence in Iowa: II. Radioactivity in Drinking Water," *American Journal of Epidemiology*, Vol. 116, No. 6, 1982b, pp. 924–932.

Beresford, S. A. A., "Cancer Incidence and Reuse of Drinking Water," *American Journal of Epidemiology*, Vol. 117, No. 3, 1983, pp. 258–268.

Black and Veatch, *Southern California Radon Survey*, prepared for Metropolitan Water District of Southern California, January 1990.

Blair, K., "Cryptosporidium and Public Health," *Health And Environment Digest*, Vol. 8, No. 8, 1994, pp. 61–65.

Blanton, M., *The Layperson's Guide to Water Recycling and Reuse*, Water Education Foundation, Sacramento, California, 1992.

Bookman-Edmonston Engineering, Inc., *Engineering Background Studies for RAND Corporation's Health Effects Study*, Glendale, California, May 1993a.

Bookman-Edmonston Engineering, Inc., *Investigation of Leaking Underground Storage Tanks in the Montebello Forebay Containing Hazardous Substances*, Glendale, California, April 1993b.

Bookman-Edmonston Engineering, Inc., "Investigation of Waste Sites in the Montebello Forebay Potentially Leaking Hazardous Substances," draft, Glendale, California, August 1993c.

Brenner, H., D. A. Savitz, K.-H. Joeckel, et al., "Effects of Nondifferential Exposure Misclassification in Ecologic Studies," *American Journal of Epidemiology*, Vol. 135, No. 1, 1992, pp. 85–95.

Brenniman, G. R., J. Vasilomanolaskis-Lagos, J. Amsel, et al., "Case-Control Study of Cancer Deaths in Illinois Communities Served by Chlorinated or Nonchlorinated Water," in R. L. Jolley, W. A. Brungs, R. B. Cumming, et al. (eds.), *Water Chlorination: Environmental Impact and Health Effects*, 3rd ed., Ann Arbor, Michigan: Ann Arbor Science Publishers, 1980, pp. 1043–1057.

Brown, H. A., "Super-chlorination at Ottumwa, Iowa," *Journal of American Water Works Association*, Vol. 32, 1940, pp. 1147–1154.

Bruvold, W. H., B. H. Olson, and M. Rigby, "Public Policy for the Use of Reclaimed Water," *Environmental Management*, Vol. 5, No. 2, 1981, pp. 95–107.

Buffler, P. A., S. P. Cooper, S. Stinnett, et al., "Air Pollution and Lung Cancer Mortality in Harris County, Texas, 1979–1981," *American Journal of Epidemiology*, Vol. 128, No. 4, 1988, pp. 683–699.

Cantor, K. P., "Water Chlorination, Mutagenicity, and Cancer Epidemiology," *American Journal of Public Health*, Vol. 84, No. 8, 1994, pp. 1211–1213.

Cantor, K. P., R. Hoover, T. J. Mason, et al., "Associations of Cancer Mortality with Halomethanes in Drinking Water," *Journal of the National Cancer Institute*, Vol. 61, No. 4, 1978, pp. 979–985.

Cantor, K. P., R. Hoover, P. Hartge, et al., "Bladder Cancer, Drinking Water Source, and Tap Water Consumption," *Journal of the National Cancer Institute*, Vol. 79, 1987, pp. 1269–1279.

Carlo, G. L., and C. J. Mettlin, "Cancer Incidence and Trihalomethane Concentration in a Public Drinking Water System," *American Journal of Public Health*, Vol. 70, No. 5, 1980, pp. 523–525.

Carpenter, L. M., and S. A. A. Beresford, "Cancer Mortality and Type of Water Source: Findings from a Study in the UK," *International Journal of Epidemiology*, Vol. 15, No. 3, 1986, pp. 312–319.

Casson, L. W., C. A. Sorber, R. H. Palmer, et al., "HIV Survivability in Wastewater," *Water Environment Research*, Vol. 64, No. 3, 1992, pp. 213–215.

CDC/ATSDR Workshop, "Use of Race and Ethnicity in Public Health Surveillance, Summary of the CDC/ATSDR Workshop," U.S. Department of Health and Human Services, *Morbidity and Mortality Weekly Report*, No. 42, 1993, pp. 1–17.

Census of Population and Housing, 1990: Summary Tape File 1 (California) [machine-readable data files]/prepared by the Bureau of the Census, Washington, DC, 1991a.

Census of Population and Housing, 1990: Summary Tape File 2 (California) [machine-readable data files]/prepared by the Bureau of the Census, Washington, DC, 1991b.

Census of Population and Housing, 1990: Summary Tape File 3 (California) [machine-readable data files]/prepared by the Bureau of the Census, Washington, DC, 1991c.

Comstock, G. W., "Water Hardness and Cardiovascular Disease," *American Journal of Epidemiology*, Vol. 110, 1979, pp. 375–400.

Cooper, C., C. A. C. Wickham, D. Barker, et al., "Water Fluoridation and Hip Fracture (letter)," *JAMA*, Vol. 266, No. 4, 1991, pp. 513–514.

Cragle, D. L., C. M. Shy, R. J. Struba, et al., "A Case-Control Study of Colon Cancer and Water Chlorination in North Carolina," in R. L. Jolley (ed.), *Water Chlorination Chemistry: Environmental Impact and Health Effects*, Chelsea, Michigan: Lewis Publishers, 1985, pp. 153–159.

Craun, G. F., *Waterborne Diseases in the US*, Boca Raton, Florida: CRC Press, Inc., 1986.

Crook, J., T. Asano, and M. Nellor, "Groundwater Recharge with Reclaimed Water in California," *Water Environment and Technology*, Vol. 2, No. 8, 1990, pp. 42–49.

Crook, J., D. K. Ammerman, D. A. Okun, and R. L. Matthews, *Guidelines for Water Reuse*, Cambridge, Massachusetts: Camp, Dresser, & McKee, 1992.

Crump, K. S., N. G. Tie-Hua, and R. G. Cuddihy, "Cancer Incidence Patterns in the Denver Metropolitan Area in Relation to the Rocky Flats Plant," *American Journal of Epidemiology*, Vol. 126, No. 1, 1987, pp. 127–135.

DeRouen, T. A., and J. E. Diem, "The New Orleans Drinking Water Controversy: A Statistical Perspective," *American Journal of Public Health*, Vol. 65, 1975, pp. 1060–1062.

DeRouen, T. A., and J. E. Diem, "Relationships Between Cancer Mortality in Louisiana Drinking Water Source and Other Possible Causative Agents," in H. H. Hiatt, J. D. Watson, and J. A. Winsten (eds.), *Origins of Human Cancer*, Vol. 4, Cold Spring Harbor Conference on Cell Proliferation, Cold Spring Harbor Laboratory, New York, 1977, pp. 331–345.

Fagliano, J., M. Berry, F. Bove, et al., "Drinking Water Contamination and the Incidence of Leukemia: An Ecologic Study," *American Journal of Public Health*, Vol. 80, No. 10, 1990, pp. 1209–1212.

Federal Register, "Rules and Regulations," Vol. 57, No. 138, July 17, 1992, p. 31778.

Federal Register, "Proposed Rules," Vol. 56, No. 138, July 18, 1991, pp. 33051–33062.

Frerichs, R. R., K. P. Satin, and E. M. Sloss, *Water Re-use: Its Epidemiologic Impact, Los Angeles County, 1969–71,* Regents of the University of California, Los Angeles, California, 1981.

Frerichs, R. R., E. M. Sloss, E. F. Maes, and K. P. Satin, *Water Re-use Part II: Its Epidemiologic Impact, Los Angeles County,* Regents of the University of California, Los Angeles, California, 1982.

Frerichs, R. R., E. M. Sloss, and E. F. Maes, *Water Re-use—Its Epidemiologic Impact Part III, Los Angeles County, 1979-80,* Regents of the University of California, Los Angeles, California, 1983.

Geschwind, S. A., J. A. J. Stolwijk, M. Bracken, et al., "Risk of Congenital Malformations Associated with Proximity to Hazardous Waste Sites," *American Journal of Epidemiology,* Vol. 135, No. 11, 1992, pp. 1197–1207.

Gottlieb, M. S., J. K. Carr, and J. R. Clarkson, "Drinking Water and Cancer in Louisiana: A Retrospective Mortality Study," *American Journal of Epidemiology,* Vol. 116, No. 4, 1982, pp. 652–667.

Gover, N., "HIV in Wastewater Not a Threat," *Water Environment Technology,* December 1993, p. 23.

Grabow, W. O. K., and M. Isaacson, "Microbiologic Quality and Epidemiological Aspects of Reclaimed Water," *Progress in Water Technology,* Vol. 10, 1978, pp. 329–335.

Greenland, S., "Divergent Biases in Ecologic and Individual-Level Studies," *Statistics in Medicine,* Vol. 11, 1992, pp. 1209–1223.

Greenland, S., and H. Morgenstern, "Ecological Bias, Confounding, and Effect Modification," *International Journal of Epidemiology,* Vol. 18, No. 1, 1989, pp. 269–274.

Griffith, J., R. C. Duncan, W. B. Riggan, et al., "Cancer Mortality in U.S. Counties with Hazardous Waste Sites and Groundwater Pollution," *Archives of Environmental Health,* Vol. 44, No. 2, 1989, pp. 69–74.

Gruener, N., *Evaluation of Toxic Effects of Organic Contaminants in Recycled Water: Final Report,* prepared for Health Effects Research Laboratory, U.S. Environmental Protection Agency, Cincinnati, Ohio, December 1978.

Hahn, R., "The State of Federal Health Statistics on Racial and Ethnic Groups," *JAMA,* Vol. 267, 1992, pp. 268–271.

Hamann, C. L., and B. McEwen, "Potable Water Reuse," in *Municipal Water Reuse: Selected Readings on Water Reuse,* Report No. EPA 430/09-91-022, United States Environmental Protection Agency, Washington, DC, September 1991, pp. 52–58.

Hatch, M. C., J. Beyea, J. W. Nieves, et al., "Cancer Near the Three Mile Island Nuclear Plant: Radiation Emissions," *American Journal of Epidemiology*, Vol. 132, No. 3, 1990, pp. 397–412.

Hatch, M. C., S. Wallenstein, J. Beyea, et al., "Cancer Rates After the Three Mile Island Nuclear Accident and Proximity of Residence to the Plant," *American Journal of Public Health*, Vol. 81, No. 6, 1991, pp. 719–724.

Herwaldt, B. L., G. F. Craun, S. L. Stokes, et al., "Waterborne Disease Outbreaks, 1989–1990," *Morbidity and Mortality Weekly Report*, Vol. 40, No. SS-3, 1991, pp. 1–21.

Higginson, J., C. S. Muir, and N. Munoz, *Human Cancer: Epidemiology and Environmental Causes*, New York: Cambridge University Press, 1992.

Hill, A. B., "The Environment and Disease: Association or Causation?" *Proceedings of the Royal Society of Medicine*, Vol. 58, 1965, pp. 295–300.

Hogan, M. D., P. Y. Chi, D. G. Hoel, et al., "Association Between Chloroform Levels in Finished Drinking Water Supplies and Various Site-Specific Cancer Mortality Rates," *Journal of Environmental Pathology and Toxicology*, Vol. 2, 1979, pp. 873–887.

Humble, C. G., and F. E. Speizer, "Polybrominated Biphenyls and Fetal Mortality in Michigan," *American Journal of Public Health*, Vol. 74, No. 10, 1984, pp. 1130–1132.

IJsselmuiden, C. B., C. Gaydos, B. Feighner, et al., "Cancer of the Pancreas and Drinking Water: A Population-Based Case-Control Study in Washington County, Maryland," *American Journal of Epidemiology*, Vol. 136, No. 7, 1992, pp. 836–842.

International Classification of Diseases, 9th Revision, Clinical Modification, 1995, Fourth Edition, Los Angeles: Practice Management Information Corporation, 1994.

Isaacson, P., J. A. Bean, R. Splinter, et al., "Drinking Water and Cancer Incidence in Iowa—III. Association of Cancer with Indices of Contamination," *American Journal of Epidemiology*, Vol. 121, No. 6, 1985, pp. 856–869.

Jablon, S., H. Zdenek, and J. D. Boice Jr., "Cancer in Populations Living Near Nuclear Facilities," *JAMA*, Vol. 265, No. 11, 1991, pp. 1403–1408.

Johnson, C. J., "Re: Cancer Incidence Patterns in the Denver Metropolitan Area in Relation to the Rocky Flats Plant," letter to the editor, *American Journal of Epidemiology*, Vol. 126, No. 1, 1987, pp. 153–155.

Kuzma, R. J., C. M. Kuzma, and C. R. Buncher, "Ohio Drinking Water Source and Cancer Rates," *American Journal of Public Health*, Vol. 67, No. 8, 1977, pp. 725–729.

Last, J. M. (ed.), *A Dictionary of Epidemiology*, New York: Oxford University Press, 1983.

Lauer, W. C., *Denver's Direct Potable Water Reuse Demonstration Project: Final Report. Executive Summary*, Denver Water Department, Denver, Colorado, April 1993.

Lawrence, C. E., P. R. Taylor, B. J. Trock, et al., "Trihalomethanes in Drinking Water and Human Colorectal Cancer," *Journal of National Cancer Institute*, Vol. 72, 1984, pp. 563–568.

Levine, W. C., W. T. Stephenson, and G. F. Craun, "Waterborne Disease Outbreaks, 1986–1988," *Morbidity and Mortality Weekly Report*, Vol. 39, No. SS-1, 1989, pp. 1–13.

Liang, K. Y., and S. L. Zeger, "Longitudinal Data Analysis Using Generalized Linear Models," *Biometrika*, Vol. 73, 1986, pp. 13–22.

Louis, M. E., "Waterborne Disease Outbreaks, 1985," *Morbidity and Mortality Weekly Report*, Vol. 37, No. SS-2, 1986, pp. 15–24.

Lynch, C. F., R. F. Woolson, T. O'Gorman, et al., "Chlorinated Drinking Water and Bladder Cancer: Effect of Misclassification on Risk Estimates," *Archives of Environmental Health*, Vol. 44, No. 4, 1989, pp. 252–259.

Mack, T. M., "Cancer Surveillance Program in Los Angeles County," *National Cancer Institute Monographs*, Vol. 47, 1977, pp. 99–101.

Marienfeld, C. J., M. Collins, H. Wright, et al., "Cancer Mortality and the Method of Chlorination of Public Drinking Water: St. Louis City and St. Louis County, Missouri," *Journal of Environmental Pathology and Toxicology*, Vol. 1, No. 1/2, 1986, pp. 141–158.

McGeehin, M. A., J. S. Reif, J. C. Becher, et al., "Case-Control Study of Bladder Cancer and Water Disinfection Methods in Colorado," *American Journal of Epidemiology*, Vol. 138, No. 7, 1993, pp. 492–501.

Metzler, D. F., R. L. Culp, H. A. Stoltenberg, et al., "Emergency Use of Reclaimed Water for Potable Supply at Chanute, Kansas," *Journal of American Water Works Association*, Vol. 50, 1958, pp. 1021–1060.

Moffa, P. E., S. D. Freedman, J. A. Hagarman, et al., "Urban Runoff and Combined Sewer Overflow," *Journal WPCF*, Vol. 55, No. 6, 1983, pp. 676–679.

Moolgavkar, S. H., "Biological Models of Carcinogenesis and Quantitative Cancer Risk Assessment," *Risk Analysis*, Vol. 14, 1994, pp. 879–886.

Morgan, H. V., memorandum to Elizabeth Sloss, "Water Quality of Domestic Supplies Served Within the Pomona Valley by the City of Pomona," March 3, 1994a.

Morgan, H. V., memorandum to Elizabeth Sloss, "Water Quality of Domestic Supplies Served Within the San Fernando Valley by the City of Los Angeles," March 3, 1994b.

Morgan, H. V., memorandum to Elizabeth Sloss, "Water Quality of Domestic Supplies Served Within the City of San Fernando," March 3, 1994c.

Moore, A. C., B. L. Herwaldt, G. F. Craun, et al., "Surveillance for Waterborne Disease Outbreaks—United States, 1991–1992," *Morbidity and Mortality Weekly Report*, Vol. 42, No. SS-5, 1993, pp. 1–22.

Moore, B. E., "Survival of Human Immunodeficiency Virus (HIV), HIV-Infected Lymphocytes, and Poliovirus in Water," *Applied and Environmental Microbiology*, Vol. 59, No. 5, 1993, pp. 1437–1443.

Morgenstern, H., "Uses of Ecologic Analysis in Epidemiologic Research," *American Journal of Public Health*, Vol. 72, No. 12, 1982, pp. 1336–1344.

Morin, M. M., A. R. Sharrett, K. R. Bailey, et al., "Drinking Water Source and Mortality in U.S. Cities," *International Journal of Epidemiology*, Vol. 14, No. 2, 1985, pp. 254–264.

Morris, R. D., A. M. Audet, I. F. Angelillo, et al., "Chlorination, Chlorination By-Products, and Cancer: A Meta-Analysis," *American Journal of Public Health*, Vol. 82, No. 7, 1992, pp. 955–963.

Nadakavukaren, A., "Water Pollution," in *Man and Environment*, Prospect Heights, Illinois: Waveland Press, Inc., 1986, pp. 327–365.

Needleman, H. L., and C. A. Gatsonis, "Low-Level Lead Exposure and IQ of Children: A Meta-Analysis of Modern Studies," *JAMA*, Vol. 263, No. 5, 1990, pp. 673–678.

Nellor, M. H., R. B. Baird, and J. R. Smyth, *Summary of Health Effects Study: Final Report*, County Sanitation Districts of Los Angeles County, Whittier, California, March 1984.

Page, T., R. H. Harris, and S. S. Epstein, "Drinking Water and Cancer Mortality in Louisiana," *Science*, Vol. 193, 1976, pp. 55–57.

Payment, P., and R. Armon, "Virus Removal by Drinking Water Treatment Processes," *Critical Reviews in Environmental Control*, Vol. 19, No. 1, 1989, pp. 15–31.

Payment, P., L. Richardson, J. Siemiatycki, et al., "A Randomized Trial to Evaluate the Risk of Gastrointestinal Disease Due to Consumption of Drinking Water Meeting Current Microbiological Standards," *American Journal of Public Health*, Vol. 81, No. 6, 1991, pp. 703–708.

Peeters, E. G., "The Influence of Soil Components and Drinking Water on the Appearance of Cancer: A Review," *Journal of Environmental Pathology, Toxicology, and Oncology*, Vol. 44, No. 4, 1992, pp. 201–204.

Polissar, L., "The Effect of Migration on Comparison of Disease Rates in Geographic Studies in the United States," *American Journal of Epidemiology*, Vol. 111, 1980, pp. 175–182.

Ram, N. M., "Environmental Significance of Trace Organic Contaminants in Drinking Water Supplies," in N. M. Ram, E. J. Calabrese, and R. F. Christman (eds.), *Organic Carcinogens in Drinking Water; Detection, Treatment, and Risk Assessment*, New York: John Wiley & Sons, 1986, pp. 3–31.

Riggs, J. L., "AIDS Transmission in Drinking Water: No Threat," *Journal of the American Water Works Association*, Vol. 81, 1989, pp. 69–70.

Robeck, G. G., K. P. Cantor, R. F. Christman, et al., *Report of the Scientific Advisory Panel on Groundwater Recharge with Reclaimed Wastewater*, prepared for State of California, State Water Resources Control Board, Department of Water Resources, Department of Health Services, November 1987.

Rothman, K. J., *Modern Epidemiology*, Boston, Massachusetts: Little, Brown and Company, , 1986.

Selvin, S., D. Merrill, L. Wong, et al., "Ecologic Regression Analysis and the Study of the Influence of Air Quality on Mortality," *Environmental Health Perspectives*, Vol. 54, 1984, pp. 333–340.

Shuval, H. I., "Direct and Indirect Wastewater Reuse for Municipal Purposes," *Ambio*, Vol. 6, 1977, pp. 63–65.

Sorlie, P., E. Backlund, and N. J. Johnson, "Mortality Among Hispanics," *JAMA*, Vol. 271, No. 16, 1994, pp. 1238–1239.

Sullivan, K., and L. Waterman, "Conference Report: Cadmium and Cancer, the Current Position. Report of an International Meeting in London, September 1988," *Annals of Occupational Hygiene*, Vol. 32, No. 4, 1988, pp. 557–560.

Swan, S. H., R. R. Neutra, M. Wrensch, et al., "Is Drinking Water Related to Spontaneous Abortion? Reviewing the Evidence from the California Department of Health Services," *Epidemiology*, Vol. 3, No. 2, 1992, pp. 83–93.

Taubes, G., "Epidemiology Faces Its Limits," *Science*, Vol. 269, 1995, pp. 164–169.

Thomas, D. C., J. Siemiatycki, R. Dewar, et al., "The Problem of Multiple Inference in Studies Designed to Generate Hypotheses," *American Journal of Epidemiology*, Vol. 122, 1985, pp. 1080–1095.

Thompson, K., R. C. Cooper, A. W. Olivieri, et al., *City of San Diego Study of Direct Potable Reuse of Reclaimed Water: Final Results*, Western Consortium for Public Health, Berkeley, California, 1992.

U.S. Environmental Protection Agency, *Drinking Water Standards and Health Advisories Table*, Washington, DC, July 1994.

Vena, J. E., S. Graham, J. Freudenheim, et al., "Drinking Water, Fluid Intake, and Bladder Cancer in Western New York," *Archives of Environmental Health*, Vol. 48, No. 3, 1993, pp. 191–197.

"Viruses and Reclaimed Water," editorial, *British Medical Journal*, Vol. 2, No. 6153, 1978, p. 1662.

Walter, S. D., "The Ecologic Method in the Study of Environmental Health. I. Overview of the Method," *Environmental Health Perspectives*, Vol. 94, 1991a, pp. 61–65.

Walter, S. D., "The Ecologic Method in the Study of Environmental Health. II. Methodologic Issues and Feasibility," *Environmental Health Perspectives*, Vol. 94, 1991b, pp. 67–73.

Wigle, D. T., Y. Mao, R. Semenciw, et al., "Contaminants in Drinking Water and Cancer Risks in Canadian Cities," *Canadian Journal of Public Health*, Vol. 77, 1986, pp. 335–342.

Wilkins, J. R., and G. W. Comstock, "Source of Drinking Water at Home and Site-Specific Cancer Incidence in Washington County, Maryland," *American Journal of Epidemiology*, Vol. 114, 1981, pp. 178–190.

Wilkins, J. R. III, N. A. Reiches, and C. W. Kruse, "Organic Chemical Contaminants in Drinking Water and Cancer," *American Journal of Epidemiology*, Vol. 110, No. 4, 1979, pp. 420–434.

World Health Organization. *Guidelines for Drinking-Water Quality*, Vol. 1, *Recommendations*, World Health Organization, Geneva, 1984.

Wrensch, M., S. H. Swan, J. Lipschomb, et al., "Spontaneous Abortions and Birth Defects Related to Tap and Bottled Water Use, San Jose, California, 1980–1985," *Epidemiology*, Vol. 3, No. 2, 1985, pp. 98–103.

Wu, M. M., T. L. Kuo, Y. H. Hwang, et al., "Dose-Response Relation Between Arsenic Concentration in Well Water and Mortality from Cancer and Vascular Diseases," *American Journal of Epidemiology*, Vol. 130, No. 6, 1989, pp. 1123–1132.

Young, T. B., M. S. Kanarek, and A. A. Tsiatis, "Epidemiologic Study of Drinking Water Chlorination and Wisconsin Female Cancer Mortality," *Journal of the National Cancer Institute*, Vol. 67, 1981, pp. 1191–1198.

Young, T. B., D. A. Wolf, and M. S. Kanarek, "Case-Control Study of Colon Cancer and Drinking Water Trihalomethanes in Wisconsin," *International Journal of Epidemiology*, Vol. 16, 1987, pp. 190–197.

Zierler, S., R. A. Danley, and L. Feingold, "Type of Disinfectant in Drinking Water and Patterns of Mortality in Massachusetts," *Environmental Health Perspectives*, Vol. 69, 1986, pp. 275–279.

Zierler, S., L. Feingold, R. A. Danley, et al., "Bladder Cancer in Massachusetts Related to Chlorinated and Chloraminated Drinking Water: A Case-Control Study," *Archives of Environmental Health*, Vol. 43, No. 2, 1988, pp. 195–200.

Zoeteman, B. C. J., "International Cooperation in Studying the Health Aspects of Organic Contaminants in Indirectly Reused Waste Water," *Annals of New York Academy of Science*, Vol. 298, 1977, pp. 561–573.

Zmirou, D., J. P. Ferley, J. F. Collin, et al., "A Follow-up Study of Gastrointestinal Diseases Related to Bacteriologically Substandard Drinking Water," *American Journal of Public Health*, Vol. 77, No. 5, 1987, pp. 582–584.